MW00359025

# Seven Sisters
## for Seven Days

*The Mothers' Manual for
Community-Based Postpartum Care*

## Michelle Peterson

Foreword by Aviva Romm, MD

Praeclarus Press, LLC
©2017 Michelle Peterson. All rights reserved.

*www.PraeclarusPress.com*

Praeclarus Press, LLC

2504 Sweetgum Lane

Amarillo, Texas 79124 USA

806-367-9950

www.PraeclarusPress.com

All rights reserved. No part of this publication may be reproduced or trans-
mitted in any form, or by any means, electronic or mechanical, including
photocopy, recording, stored in a database, or any information storage, or
put into a computer, without the prior written permission from the publisher.

**DISCLAIMER**

The information contained in this publication is advisory only and is not
intended to replace sound clinical judgment or individualized patient care.
The author disclaims all warranties, whether expressed or implied, including
any warranty as the quality, accuracy, safety, or suitability of this information for any particular purpose.

ISBN: 978-1-939807-89-2

©2017 Michelle Peterson. All rights reserved.

Cover Design: Ken Tackett
Cover Illustration: Tamara Adams
Developmental Editing: Kathleen Kendall-Tackett
Copy Editing: Chris Tackett
Layout & Design: Nelly Murariu

*Dedicated to my mother, my forever friend and listening ear. Thank you for teaching me about love, kindness, compassion, and strength.*

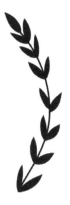

# MORE ADVANCED PRAISE

"Birth preparation in today's world often neglects the most important issue imaginable ... becoming a mother! Somehow we presume that once the baby is born that all the hard work is done... when in truth the work has only begun. Michelle's book, Seven Sisters for Seven Days unfolds the truth of what is missing in our society, and shines a light on a path which will renew a new mother's joy in motherhood."

—LYNN BAPTISTI RICHARDS,
midwife & author of *The Vaginal Birth
After Cesarean (VBAC) Experience:
Birth Stories by Parents and Professionals*

"Please pick up this book and nourish a new mom. Please bring this book into your community through your midwifery or doula practice. Please start food trees and have honest conversations over tea with new moms. Each of us needs to know we are not alone."

—AVIVA ROMM,
MD, author of *The Natural Pregnancy Book,
Natural Health After Birth, Botanical Medicine for
Women's Health,* and *The Adrenal Thyroid Revolution*

# CONTENTS

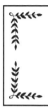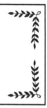

# ACKNOWLEDGEMENTS

To all the women in my life who believed in this vision, recognized the importance of it, supported our family through many births, and helped me to find the courage to share this program, I say thank you. Jenn Marie & Chocolatree Organic Eatery, Shama, Tara, Jess, Kayt, Lucy, Sunny, Tiffany, Sarah, KC, Zoe, Shell, Lynn, Danielle, Rachel, Midwives Rising, Peaches, Stephanie, Annie, Laura, Bernadette, Alicia, Andrea, Ysha Oakes and the Sacred Window School, Lorna, all the Seven Sisters Facilitators, this program could not have been born without your inspiration and support.

Mom and Dad you have always believed in me, always supported my endeavors, and have been constant cheer leaders for this project. Thank you for your never-ending love not to mention help with the boys while I finished this book. Thank you to my entire Peterson family and extended family for your support and cheerleading.

Stephanie, Nona, Celeste, & James thank you for your love, many hours of playing with the boys while I wrote, and for being in our lives and for all your support!

To the mentor midwives in my life; Shell Walker Luttrell you have been a midwife, mentor, role model, and guide for this entire project. Thank you for your faith, encouragement, and for midwifing the title of the book! Lynn Baptisti Richards, you have always been an ear, a voice of wisdom, and guide. Thank you.

Frank Oliveira, you have been a constant support, an angel on earth. The lessons you have taught me are invaluable, and I will carry them through my life and intend on sharing them with many others. Thank you.

Thank you to all the ladies who submitted stories, pictures, and art. La Pachanga Photography & Jennifer Lind Schutsky for your beautiful images, Tamara Adams for your perfect cover art, and Rael, Leela, Annie, Danielle, Sarah Carter, Lynn Baptisti Richards, and Shell Walker Luttrell for your personal submissions.

To the women who supported me in my first postpartum in the way of your insightful works in the world, Robin Lim, Ina May Gaskin, Aviva Romm, thank you for your wisdom and inspiration.

Kathleen Kendall-Tackett and Praeclarus Press, thank you for being so wonderful to work with and for believing in this book!

Clint, we have been on quite the journey, and I have learned so much beside you as we walk together as partners and parents. Thank you for your spiritual walk of life, editorial insights, and for being there for the boys and I in the many ways that you are.

Most of all, thank you to my boys, who have taught me (and continue to teach me) about how deep love can go, what I am capable of, and have given the opportunity to experience unconditional love. It's through loving you I have learned how to love myself better.

Thank you!

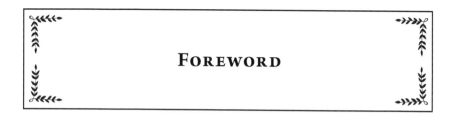

# FOREWORD

The transition to new motherhood is complex, overwhelming, and can feel like nothing short of a near vertical mountain climb for many women. And yes, it is often beautiful. But even that, not for every woman. We are shifting at every level – our physical body down to our cells, and then more obviously, our sleep (or lack thereof) and lifestyle patterns, even our core identity. It can be hard. Really hard. I have four kids. Been there, done that. I know. I've also assisted thousands of women through their births and through my books, and have seen and heard stories of the highs – and the lows.

Yet the reality of how hard the transition to new motherhood can be is often under acknowledged, both by women as we worry whether expressing our true feelings and needs would somehow suggest we are "good enough moms," as if struggling means that "Being a mother just doesn't come naturally to me" or worse, that we secretly don't love being a mom, and by societal norms that expect us to be back on our feet and back to work within 6 weeks, with feeding, childcare, and our emotional needs and those of our new baby all figured out.

And how's that going for us? Not so well, it seems, given high rates of overwhelming exhaustion, and frustration at the least, and postpartum depression for many, and some of the tragedies we read about in the news at the hands of a new mother at the other end of the spectrum.

Yet the science is clear: having attentive, caring support – an extra pair of hands, some cooked meals, and understanding can make this transition if not always easy breezy, healthy, and even joyful. We are meant to raise children in community, not in the isolation so many of us experience as new mothers. Having baskets of fresh-made food brought to me so that my partner, who didn't have paternity leave and was trying to juggle being a new dad (and as we had more kids, take care of them so I could take care of baby) could stress-less, having friends pick up my older kids so I could take a nap with baby, and having loving hands take care of new baby so I could eat and shower – these simple things – can feel like – and may even be – a lifesaver.

I couldn't be more proud of Michelle's book and community-based postpartum care program. I've watched this program evolve from her first questions to me. "Do you think this is a good idea? Do you think there's a need?" And as I said to her then, I am saying to you, "YES. YES. YES." Please pick up this book and nourish a new mom. Please bring this book into your community through your midwifery or doula practice. Please start food trees and have honest conversations over tea with new moms. Each of us needs to know we are not alone. As we mother and love our children, isn't this one of the core beliefs we deeply desire to pass on with every kiss, every time baby is at breast, every snuggle, kissed booboo, and every tear they shed? So too, we need to know we are not alone in the intense job of becoming a mother, being a mother, and staying yourself, intact, healthy, and whole. Consciously creating your new momma plan is as important as thinking about what you will eat during your pregnancy, where and with whom you will birth. As you learn to give as a mom, learn to receive as women – the help that will make the mom journey so much more fun, easier, more honest and sane, and when it's your turn, pass that on to the next momma. And so community begins.

With love,

Aviva Romm, MD, midwife, herbalist

September 14, 2016

Author of *The Natural Pregnancy Book, Natural Health After Birth, Botanical Medicine for Women's Health,* and *The Adrenal Thyroid Revolution.*

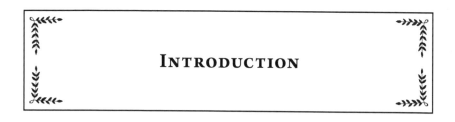

# INTRODUCTION

This book started writing itself in my heart during my first postpartum period, wherein I gathered an understanding of the many hills and valleys a mother is asked to climb and traverse. Like many new mothers, I had no idea what was going to be asked of me as I became a mother. I learned not only what my limitations were, but also my strengths. I learned what loving another as much as I love my sons does to a woman's heart; she walks around with it wide open, feeling the world with a compassionate embrace. I also learned how much support I really needed, that I did not choose to do this alone, and that I ached for a community to hold me as I came to discover how to not only care for my child, but also myself. My children and my family asked for all of me, and I choose to show up fully.

Becoming a new mother unraveled every part of me, and I put myself back together as I became the new woman I was walking in the world. When my second child arrived, it was my sacred duty to set myself up with comprehensive postpartum care out of love for my entire family, knowing that if this mama has a full cup, she can show up to her role with everything she has. And I did, with all the support in the world.

Many opportunities for growth drop themselves at your door when you become a mother, and when a new being enters your life. For new mothers, many of these initiations are inherent, natural, and necessary. However, there are also experiences, such as isolation, fear, depression, and lack of compassionate care, that is most certainly not natural and necessary for our mothers. This book, and this program, is offered to the community of mothers out of a clear need for more postpartum support. I set it up with the intention of getting mothers more comprehensive, compassionate, community postpartum care. My heart shares it with the hope that we continue to pass it on, recognize the value of our mothers, and recognize how this care ripples down to our children and our communities.

A nurtured mother yields a full cup that is able to pour gracefully into the hearts and hands of the children and family she feeds with every part of her. This love pours from infinite spaces within the mother. Imagine now, that we care for her, as we would care for a tree that bears much fruit every single year. We value that fruit-bearing tree, whose bounty nourishes us, and we understand the importance of caring for it. Let us nourish our mother, as we nourish that tree, or that business, or that project we are so invested in. A nourished mother is an investment. She pours her love and her being onto the family, her relationships, into the food she cooks, and the milk she makes, either with her own body or through preparation. She tends to her home, or the work she does in the world to keep the home warm, however she expresses herself. That love she pours into her family is gold, pure nourishment, and it feeds many. A nurtured mother is an investment we all would benefit from. Not only does this fill her reserves, but it benefits her children, family, relationships, and community. Let us see the value in taking good care of our mothers, an investment that will pay off in dividends for all of us.

*You there*

*Made of clay*

*Sweet breath*

*Simple heat*

*And the sacred ash of 8 billion fallen stars...*

*Know this*

*Claim this*

*Let it reverberate through the celestial cosmos of your soul and the silvery black shiny depths of your heavenly design*

*You are the truth.*

*There is nothing less*

*Nothing more*

*There is always something more*

*You hold eternity in your arms*

*You are cradled in our arms*

*You are not alone.*

*©Shell Walker Luttrell, Midwife*

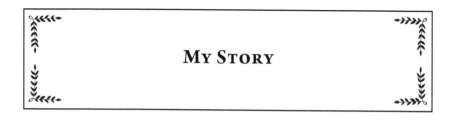

# MY STORY

I am a mother. Affectionately called Mama Bear by my friends, I have always been instinctively propelled towards caring for the needs of others. I became happily pregnant in 2010 with our first son, and thus began my true journey into motherhood. My husband and I chose to do a homebirth and hired a licensed midwife whom we both resonated with and trusted. My pregnancy was physically uneventful. I ate everything in sight, it seemed, and did not think much about it. I loved being pregnant. My pregnancy was a very spiritual journey for me and our son's birth was no different. I felt surrounded by all the women in the world and guided by a benevolent presence throughout. I planned for months for my birth, set up a gorgeous birth room, and it set the stage for what was a powerful vision quest for me.

During labor, I went deep into meditation, and it was an intense, painful, and powerful experience. When my son finally arrived into my arms, it zapped me back to earth naturally, as I held him. I remember I kept saying, "I just need a few minutes to take this in." I held my beautiful boy in my arms, and slowly moved to a couch to be fed by our beautiful birth assistant, and to regain my strength. I felt dizzy, exhausted, confused, all the while completely in love, and elated. I remember my arms shaking, and the anxiety at feeling as if I could not hold my baby because I was exhausted and depleted. In the days that followed, my son did not sleep well, and I had many sleepless nights myself. I had it in my head that I had to stop any cry that ever erupted from him, and would wear him constantly in the baby carrier. He did not like to sleep unless he was attached to me, and if I tried to put him down, he would wake up. Thus began the voyage of bouncing around the house at all hours of the night with my wee one. The love I had for him scared me, healed me, opened me up, and it invited emotional whirlwinds.

15

In the days that followed, I had friends come and go with food, and my husband soon went back to work for long days. Yet still, I had very little postpartum care, and by week 2, I felt very much on my own. It was hard to even make food because I was often bouncing around the house while wearing my baby. I did not ask for help because I did not think I was supposed to. I also had a hard time receiving help. I thought this was just how it was. My mother did it this way, so I assumed other mothers did it, and I could do it too. I am a mother; this is what I am supposed to do. Somewhere, I decided I was supposed to be a superwoman, but later, I realized I did not have to be.

I spent many days alone in that house, or walking through the neighborhood with my sweet little babe. I did not have television or movies. I had books, and books I did read when I could. My midwife lent me *After the Baby's Birth* by Robin Lim, which I hardly even looked at until, wouldn't you know, after my baby's birth. This book opened my eyes to much of what I created after the birth of my second son, but more on that later.

Months into my postpartum period, I got increasingly tired, I could not think straight, and I was starting to feel blue. I loved my baby, and I did not understand how I could feel so much love and so much confusion all at once. I kept writing it off to "this is how it is" because of lack of sleep. I went for over a year like this before I decided I had better get a deeper check-up and blood work. I opened up to my naturopathic doctor and we ran tests, and recognized I had a lot going on. My body was deeply depleted, my thyroid was underactive, my adrenals were shot, and I had leaky gut, all going on at once. With the help of my doctor, I went on an intensive herbal protocol for my adrenals, as well as thyroid support to help support my body.

Once I was done breastfeeding, we went deeper into my healing and I went on for 3 years bringing my body back into balance. During the coming years, I also studied postpartum practices, such as Ayurvedic postpartum care, holistic midwifery, herbs for the postpartum, as well as postpartum care practices in other cultures. I became passionate about supporting other mothers and created community support networks, meal trains for new mothers, as well as weekly mothers' groups with guest speakers speaking on topics to support mothers and families. I knew it did not have to be so hard on our mothers.

Three years later, when my husband and I decided to conceive our second child, I spent my entire pregnancy planning for the postpartum. I called upon all the resources I had built over the years, and planned what I called my postpartum protocol. This protocol involved a postpartum Ayurvedic-inspired meal menu, which I created with the help of Ysha Oakes' *Postpartum Ayurvedic Cookbook*. I created an herbal regimen, in the form of teas, with the help of an herbalist and my naturopath. I put a mother-warming protocol in place, and made sure to have items to keep myself warm, such as warm socks and a kidney/belly wrap. We also hired the most incredible midwife and team ever, who were an amazing resource and support in the postpartum. I hired a postpartum doula, only to find out 2 months later that she was pregnant. I had to come up with something else, so being the creative woman that I am, I called upon my friends to help me.

I had many friends offering help to our family in the postpartum period. I was amazed by it, so I asked them, instead of baby gifts, if they would love to give the gift of their time. I wrote a letter, which asked for this help, and asked people only to volunteer if they had the time, to volunteer skills they loved to do, and only do it if they loved doing it. I would only feel good about receiving that help if it came in a balanced way, and come forward did my sisters ever!

One of my dear sisters owns a restaurant and offered to make my postpartum meals as a special addition in her restaurant, and would deliver them by the gallon. I showed her my postpartum cookbook and she went to work, even consulting with an Ayurvedic doctor. I was blown away by her support. She and I sat in my house one afternoon and came up with "The Seven Sisters" name. This postpartum meal was even offered as a special to the community with a discount to postpartum women. This is where the Seven Sisters was gestated, out of a desire to support my family and myself in the postpartum period so I would not crash as I did with my first. I chose to be there full force for my babies, myself, and my relationship. I knew if I got this support for my body and being, I would not go energetically bankrupt like I did the first time. I knew the importance of it. I loved myself enough to ask for it.

My second son's birth was very different from my first. It was fast and intense. I was very much in my body. Something deep and ancient healed inside of me that night, and that is between the Creator and me, but it was profound. The Seven Sisters Team was born and activated. Meals started coming by the gallon every couple of days. I consumed dahls, porridges, and warming meals. I drank warm teas morning and night. I wrapped my kidneys and kept my feet warm. I hardly left my bed unless I had to. My little guy and I snuggled and integrated. It was such a sweet and beautiful time together. I felt nourished, cared for, and supported. Women did not often come into our home, but would drop things off, and most days', women were just on call and did not come, but just knowing they were there was the support I needed.

I had particularly painful afterbirth pains and contractions, and was highly emotional and letting go of a lot. I do believe my son helped guide the creation of this care as well as my inner knowing, because I really needed this window to heal and integrate. My sisters came and did my laundry, played with my other son, fed me meals, cleaned my house, or just talked with me with sweet presence. It was one of the most healing experiences of my life, one that I will *never* forget. I felt more in balance in the following weeks than I had experienced in a long time. I had energy, my mind was clear, my heart was full, and my being nurtured deeply. It was a notable difference to not only myself, but also those around me. My thyroid levels had stabilized, my gut and digestion were in prime shape, and it was truly a healing sacred window.

I know that the Seven Sisters Support contributed to my profoundly different second postpartum, and I believe that any mother, no matter what her circumstances, can create some level of support to accompany her lifestyle. It is important that we value the care of mothers, not only as a society, but also as mothers, that we recognize the necessity for proper self-care and its implications for the entire familial unit and beyond.

Mothers, my message to you is this: understand what you need as a mother and woman to thrive. Identify for yourself and your family how you can be best cared for so you have all the resources to draw upon to care for them. You have plenty of time to do it all; trust me, you will. Take this time, at one of the most vulnerable times in your life, to receive the care you deserve. You, your children, and your relationship will all benefit from it. Other mothers will benefit as well, seeing that, yes, mothers are valuable, and yes, we must nurture and care for the mother.

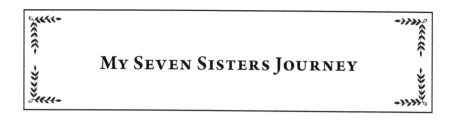

# MY SEVEN SISTERS JOURNEY

Most of us no longer live in communities or tribes, so sometimes a family will hire a postpartum doula to live with them and support the family unit in the postpartum period. This is a beautiful service, yet not all women will acquire it, and many women I know crave the encouraging comfort of friends and family during this special time.

This is the very thing I have done: I asked my community to support our family in the postpartum period. Some may think I did this purely as an act of self-love, and yes that is definitely part of it, but the most prominent driving force for me was knowing that I needed support to maintain my health and balance that I worked so diligently on after the birth of our first son to fully show up for my family.

When we received the care of the Seven Sisters Program, I did not realize the amount of impact it would have on my heart and soul. We received support in the way of childcare, meals, a team on-call each day for 6 weeks, people caring for our horses, and even the loaning of cars and rides when our car was at the mechanic before the birth to get us to the midwife. Each person contributed in some way to bringing ease to our family as we prepared for our little arrival. This allowed us to prepare emotionally, together without pressure, stress, and fear. On the deepest level, it taught me how to receive love and support, something that has not been easy for me to receive, although I freely give it.

Our team gave us the gift of unconditional support, a gift that I will carry into all my relationships as I endeavor to support my family, friends, and community. Receiving this contribution from our community, reaping the incredible rewards, and seeing how deeply it can serve others, was the seed from which the program was born.

## CHAPTER 1

# THE IMPORTANCE OF POSTPARTUM CARE

*"Is ours not a strange culture that focuses so much attention on childbirth—virtually all of it based on anxiety and fear—and so little on the crucial time after birth, when patterns are established that will affect the individual and the family for decades?"*

SUZANNE ARMS

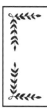
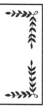
# WHAT WE NEED AS MOTHERS

**Lynn Baptisti Richards**

What we need as mothers is the same as what every human needs, such as love, and food for the body, mind, heart, and soul. Imagine yourself being told since the time you were very young that you will have a role to play in the history of humankind; that this is what you were born to do, and that there is nothing more important in this life than your success in doing this one amazingly important thing. Imagine that this message is repeated to you over time, as you are growing up. But no one ever tells you what you are going to need to know in order to succeed. In fact, when you ask about it, they tell you that there is nothing anyone can ever tell you to prepare you for this job. There are no words to describe it. But somehow, you will be expected to know what to do when you get there.

You will be expected to do this alone. Your hours will be 24/7, 365 days a year, for a lifetime. You will never have a day off, and you will receive absolutely no financial compensation. However, somehow, you will also be expected to make the money you need in order to do this monumentally important job. You will be held responsible for the entire life of at least one other human being, or perhaps many. But you will be given very little credit, and will most likely be blamed by the ones who have been in your care. And if you fail at this job, your heart will be broken in ways that you can never imagine.

These are the messages that many girls are given about becoming mothers. Strangely enough, it's actually the truth!

Is there any wonder that most young women walk into motherhood ill-prepared, ridden with anxiety, and fearful of asking for the help they need?

In other societies, in days gone by, families lived close together. Extended families, tribes, and communities knew that the babies were the most important assets that could possibly be obtained. In today's world, babies are expenditures. This basic conceptual change explains all the problems of young mothers of today.

Our society is having a postpartum hemorrhage! Women are bleeding out! Their entire life force is leaving. It is silent. Apparently, no one is suffering. But if we don't recognize the problem, and take action, the children will grow up motherless.

Back in the 70s, women had a revolution! We wanted to be equal to men. We wanted to be doctors, lawyers, accountants, and executives. We were tired of being second-class citizens. We were tired of being afraid that we could not take care of ourselves and our babies. We burned our bras, and wrote treatises about how much a wife is worth. We thought that having jobs would bring us the respect we were lacking. But we were wrong.

What women really need is the same thing we have all always needed: to be loved and respected for doing our most important work, which is the work that will sustain an entire society for generations to come, for being mothers. I have no idea when, or in what society, women were actually loved and respected for being mothers. I hope there actually was at least one society that held motherhood as the most honorable work possible. Unfortunately, I doubt that that was ever actually true. I think we like to imagine that there was a tribe somewhere in the world, at some time in history that held mothers as equal to warriors or kings.

If not, well, let's imagine it so. Let's imagine that in our society, in this time in history, a sudden revolution has occurred as a great revelation from God, in all the religions of the world that proclaimed the elevation of the status of mothers to near godliness. Indeed, how then would a new mother be treated by her husband, her family, her friends, her workplace, and her community?

Let's imagine the story of the birth of Jesus. Three kings arrived bearing gifts. Imagine a king (or queen) coming to the bedside of every new mother, bearing gifts that would aid in the health and well-being of the baby and the mother? Imagine the "king of the workplace" offering to give the money needed to support the family for those first few crucial months, so that no mother would be forced to leave her tiny baby to return to her work on an assembly line? Imagine angels coming. Perhaps they might bring food, hands to help in the kitchen, or caring for the other children, or even to draw the mother a bath, and give her a much-deserved massage? Imagine the wise women coming; the older ones who have been down the path of motherhood, to help when the baby was crying, or the mother's breasts were sore. Imagine that no one feared to offer, and no one feared to ask for the help that all mothers need and deserve.

We know that in other countries, there are paid professional doulas, trained and paid by the government, to attend to women postpartum in their homes. We know that in other countries, midwives attend the births of women in their own homes, and continue their work after the birth with at least weekly, and often-times daily, visits to the mothers in their own homes. We do know that in other countries, all medical care is provided to mothers and babies as a human right, and no one need fear the cost of medical care as a deterrent from getting good care. We do know that in other countries, mothers and fathers receive paid family leave for up to 2 years after a baby is born. We know that it is possible to stop the postpartum hemorrhage!

We can do this one person at a time for one mother at a time. We can make a change from within ourselves. We can honor every mother as she passes us at the grocery store. Just the very inner change of thought can transmit through the wall of silence. For every new mother we know, we can step forward and offer ourselves in whatever manner we can serve best. We can become political. We can organize our own communities. We can take action.

Most importantly, we can listen to what new mothers are saying. We can listen with an open heart. Take mothers out of solitary confinement! Become a mother's confidant. Of all the gifts, of all the services, of all the work we can do for new mothers, what a new mother needs most is a sister, a friend, or a mother to mother her through her labor of love of becoming a new mother.

Although being a mother is never completed, it is at the beginning that we grow our roots. It is at the beginning that we are pushing up the ground from beneath, as we are lifting our heads to unfurl into becoming the new being we ourselves are creating; ourselves as mothers. Not only do we have a new baby to care for, but we ourselves are becoming a new being. Becoming a mother is a powerful and arduous journey. When we become a mother, we officially leave our carefree little girl behind. This is not done without pain or confusion or wistful longing. We will, one day, have time again for ourselves. But we will never again be the same self we gave up the day we became a mother. And there is grief for what has been lost. That journey through the loss deserves compassion. We, who have the opportunity to support a new young mother on her journey need to remember to listen to her story and love her. The truer the love, compassion, and support she receives, the smoother her transition into motherhood will be.

We cannot, and should never aspire to, take away anything from her experience. We cannot take the bumps out of the road. We can suggest a different path. But she must choose her own. She is on a journey of her own making. We are along for the ride.

Imagine she is learning to ride a bike. It is true that there is nothing anyone can do or say to teach someone how to ride a bike. We cannot ride it for her. She does have to learn to do it for herself. But we can run alongside of her. We can shout words of enthusiasm. We are there to pick her up when she loses her balance and scrapes her knees. We are there to shout for joy when she realizes that she's finally got it!

The very best things we learn in life don't come from books, or the Internet, or even from our best friends. We don't learn the best stuff in school. And we certainly can't take an exam to prove we know all the best stuff to be certified as a "stuff knower." The best stuff that we learn in life, we learn from inside ourselves. We have an inner knowing. The trick is to find the path that will allow us to access that inner knowing.

Most of the time, that path has something to do with getting stuff out of the way, more than it does with accumulating more information. So when we feel confused in our learning about becoming a new mother, stop, take a breath, take as long a breath as you can possibly take, and let it out really, really slowly, and ask, "How can I get out of my own way right now?" It's the single most important question to ask. If you are the friend, or sister, or support person, ask yourself the exact same question, because if our stuff is in the way, we can't help anyone else at all. **Clearing the path, alone and together. That is the best postpartum support ever!**

LYNN BAPTISTI RICHARDS was a pioneer midwife during the resurgence of midwifery of the 70s and 80s. She practiced for more than 20 years, and attended more than 1000 births. Her calling to the practice of midwifery began with the birth of her first baby in 1975, an unnecessary and life-changing cesarean. Her next baby, born in 1978, was one of the first VBACs in this country. Shortly thereafter, she started the first VBAC classes, before the term VBAC had ever been coined. After completing her midwifery training, she devoted most of her practice to VBAC mothers, and to other mothers who had had prior traumatic births. Her first book, *The Vaginal Birth After Cesarean Experience—Very Beautiful and Courageous,* was published in 1987, after which she taught workshops and gave lectures on VBAC throughout the English-speaking world. Today, she continues to write and teach, while attending to her greatest gift: her grandchildren.

# HEARTFELT SHARING FROM A POSTPARTUM DOULA AND MOTHER

## Annie S., Mother and Birth and Postpartum Caregiver

As a doula and a mother, I have been on both ends of postpartum and now, more than ever, recognize on such a deep level the importance of this sacred time for a woman. It was always a pleasure and such a joy to tend to the new family; to witness the growth and magic that a new human brings to those around; to watch this new life open more and more, just like a delicate flower, every day and witness the love that radiates from the budding family's hearts. It has always been a passion of mine to nurture, and when I discovered postpartum care, never more had this passion been so fed by my awareness of what could be some of the most critical days of a mother's life. I knew I was doing something important, and it was not until my son was born that the importance hit on a new level. When I received postpartum care, I recognized what I was doing for women.

The postpartum is a time for bonds to be made, for healing to take place, for recapitulations of birthing (which can be very emotional), for families to find new rhythms, for a mother to rebuild her cellular make up from the ground up, and for so much unseen work between a mother and child. In addition, for me, it did not matter how great or how small any action was. The love with which someone swept the dust from under the table because I could see it from where I was laying everyday with my baby was felt. It was the same when my best friend, in her postpartum, asked me to hang her clothes in color order because that is what she noticed as she lay in her bed with her new one, day in and day out. We do these things for new mothers because we care. We want mothers to feel completely saturated in love and care, so that when 40 days rolls around, and the sisters come around less and less for the tidying and cooking, that mother feels cared for. She feels restored. She feels ready to enter back into her role in her family. That mother will be more capable, more patient, and more willing, and so it is feeding the future of the world.

As a postpartum doula, I really want to know what you need to feel completely at peace in your home, even if it's the way that the dishes are put away, or the order in which your clothes are hung in your closet. There is a special fluffing of the heart that comes about serving a mother. Maybe it's the feeling of serving The Mother of All That Is. As I get on my knees to reach that dust bunny far beneath the couch, I am on my knees to the Mother of All of Us, thanking her for this new life and the life of this mother.

So mothers, ask for what you need. Ask for what you want. Your family and friends are here to serve you.

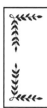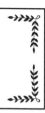

# THE IMPORTANCE OF
# POSTPARTUM CARE

There has been a growing awareness in recent years around the challenges that new mothers face in the Western world. According to the World Health Organization, about 10% of Western pregnant women, and 13% of women who have just given birth experience a mental disorder, primarily depression. Up to 80% of women experience some kind of "baby blues" in the first 6 weeks after the birth of their baby.

> As citizens of an industrialized nation, we often act as if we have nothing to learn from the Third World. Yet many of these cultures are doing something extraordinarily right–especially, in how they care for new mothers. In their classic paper, Stern and Kruckman (1983) present an anthropological critique of the literature. They found that in the cultures they studied, postpartum disorders, including the "baby blues," were virtually non-existent. In contrast, 50% to 85% of new mothers in industrialized nations experience the "baby blues," and 15% to 25% (or more) experience postpartum depression. What makes the difference? Stern and Kruckman noted that cultures who had low incidence of postpartum mood disorders all had rituals that provided support and care for new mothers.

> KATHLEEN KENDALL-TACKETT

Before I had a baby, and even during my pregnancy, I did not think of the postpartum beyond preparing for our baby, nor did I recognize it as a period in time that one would prepare for, or think that there was any cultural significance attached to it. This simply was not talked about by any of the women in my life. You had the baby, and that was that. This is common for many women in Western culture. New mothers do not realize what their postpartum needs are until after the baby arrives, and tasks that were previously easy to handle become overwhelming. The focus is placed primarily on the arriving baby and the birth, not on the mother after the baby arrives. After the baby's birth is precisely the time when a mother and family require loving care and support from their community. This can be accomplished through creating a supportive postpartum protocol and care network that allows the new familial unit to have a gentle integration.

A new mother shares her journey with the postpartum period with very little planning beyond getting ready for the baby:

> As for postpartum support, I thought, no big deal, my husband can take as much time off as needed to help. It is just caring for a little baby, after all. Nursing, changing diapers, how could it be too hard? Well, I did not anticipate how, in spite of having a natural birth at home, I would not be able to sit for about 3 days because of being so swollen, and that I would not really feel somewhat normal walking around for about a week. My entire body was so sore from the physical exertion of labor, I felt like I had participated in a triathlon without any training. I also did not anticipate things like uterine prolapse and terrible hemorrhoids, and how it is better to not walk around much, or even wear your baby in a sling for the first 6 weeks, or so if this is something you are healing from. I did not realize how weird my abdomen would look and feel after giving birth and my organs slowly moving back into place again. It was literally the hardest work I had done in my life. I did not realize I would then only sleep a couple of hours each night the next 5 days or so. Although I did not anticipate it, I would have loved to have a woman clean up after the birth, do a load of laundry, and cook us a meal so we could just rest with our baby after he was born.

> LEELA, NEW MOTHER

The lack of knowledge about the postpartum period leaves many women unprepared and overwhelmed when their baby arrives. They have the nursery, baby clothes, baby monitor, nursing bras, breast pump, or whatever else they choose for their baby, but they are possibly left with sore bottoms, leaky breasts, an overwhelmed psyche, expanded heart, and, often, very little tools beyond the love for their child to manage it all—and for many with very little help. This is not to say all women have this experience, thankfully there are also many women who have families and friends who understand what the postpartum is like, and show up to support them. Awareness around more adequate postpartum care is becoming more and more common in our country. Light is now being shed on postpartum depression through stars in the media coming forward speaking to their own challenges. One television star, Hayden Panettiere, spoke out on postpartum depression in the name of supporting new mothers.

> When [you are told] about postpartum depression you think it's, "I feel negative feelings towards my child. I want to injure or hurt my child." I've never, ever had those feelings. Some women do. But you don't realize how broad of a spectrum you can really experience that on. It's something that needs to be talked about. Women need to know that they're not alone, and that it does heal.

> HAYDEN PANETTIERE

We live in a culture that often glorifies stars, and because a star experienced depression, and spoke out about it, it drew coverage and attention. American cities are now exploring paid parental leave, and there has been talk of this in New York, California, and beyond. People are waking up to the fact that this is a problem in our society. This is a step in the right direction. Through recognizing there is a problem, we can start implementing solutions.

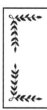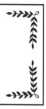

# POSTPARTUM PRACTICES IN OTHER CULTURES

We live in a culture bereft of ritual around both childbirth and the post-partum period. This leaves women often feeling isolated, disconnected from community, and unclear on how to adapt to their newly emerging role in the world with very little tools and guideposts to help navigate it.

> In the traditional non-Western view, birth is part of a holistic and personal system, involving moral values, social relations, and relation to the environment, as well as the physical aspects. Birth ceremonies often are used to recognize the importance of the event in the culture [Leininger, et. al (1995) cited by Yeoun Soo Kim-Godwin (2003)].

In many non-Western cultures, there are also specific practices for the post-partum period, such as lying in, also referred to as confinement, keeping the mother warm and/or mother roasting, special diets, as well as rituals and ceremonies. Many cultures have this window of time in which the mother (and sometimes the partner) lays in with the baby in the name of recuperation, healing, as well as honoring cultural norms and beliefs for some.

> In almost all non-Western societies, 40 days after birth is seen as necessary for recuperation. Among most non-Western cultures, family members (especially female relatives) provide strong social support; help new mothers at home during that period. The new mother's activities are strictly limited, and her needs are taken care of by (typically) female relatives and midwives (Holroyd et al., 1997; Nahas & Amashen, 1999 cited by Yeoun Soo Kim-Godwin, 2003).

> The majority of the births in Holland take place at home. Excellent in-home postpartum care is provided by women

called *Kraamverpleegsters* (professional maternity nurse). They arrive at 8 a.m. and leave at 5 p.m. for 8 days. These angels take care of the laundry, cooking, shopping, child-care, and act as hostess for visitors, and do postpartum check-ups as well. They have daily contact with the midwife or doctors who attended the birth, reporting all progress of the mother and baby. Infant care is provided, parenting skills are taught, and breastfeeding is supported

ROBIN LIM

Postpartum care practices are carried out in other cultures with an under-standing that the postnatal family is in a vulnerable state and require additional support. When we value not only our mothers, but also our growing families, we recognize the cultural importance of mothering our mothers in the name of nurtured families and communities. This is the goal and intention of the Seven Sisters Program: to nurture mothers, families, and the global community.

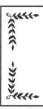
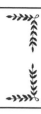

# MOTHERING OUR MOTHERS

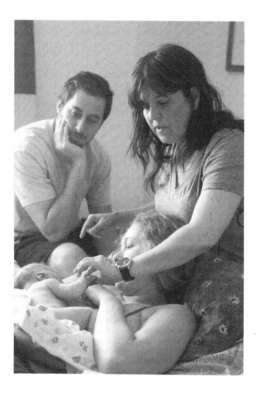

Motherhood is also the essence of people taking care of people. Without this, culture itself dries up, leaving our children and ourselves without roots. When any culture allows its women to lose their health and joy through the process of re-creation, people lose touch with the greatest source of its natural enfoldment of lovingness, its vitality, and its innate mappings back "home." It is essential on so many levels, and especially potent in the postnatal time, that we support Mothers to feel at home within themselves.

YSHA OAKES

During my first pregnancy, no one really talked with me about the post-partum period. I did not think of much beyond having a comfortable nightie. I did not know who my breastfeeding counselors were—or that they even existed. Nor did I know what complications could arise during breast-feeding. It is just how it was. I had breastfeeding issues come up and had no idea where to turn. I suffered silently for a solid week until I realized some-thing was not right. My midwife, after receiving many concerning calls from me, connected me with a La Leche League leader, who I talked with over the phone. She was able to identify that it may be my baby's latch. She could not come see me because of her busy schedule and there were no other consul-tants in our area. With a breastfeeding book, I did my research, worked on my little boy's latch, and we finally found our way.

It was not easy, and now I know I did not have to suffer as much as I did. I remember, later into my postpartum, when I spoke to other mothers in the community, that many others were struggling just as I was. They felt that this was just how it was. They did not know what to ask for either, and were frustrated by what felt like a lack of support systems available. We found ways to gather and support each other, but sometimes, it just seemed like too much for a mother to even do that. One mother reported to me, in the grocery store, that she did not make it to a lot of our events because it was just too challenging managing the two kids on her own.

Then I became that mother. I hiked all over the valley with my first child in the carrier on my own. But with two, it is a very different picture. Yes, there are ways to make it happen, and I am an innovative woman, and I make my hikes still happen. But the thought of managing two kids on a trail is a daunting task on some days. Even going to the grocery store can be. I do it, and we all survive just fine. However, the point I am trying to make, is the distinct overwhelm that happens when you feel like you are doing it on your own. This, I feel, is a big contributor to depression, isolation, and anxiety in mothers.

I can speak from personal experience, when my second son was only a few months old, going through a day when I knew my husband would not be home until 9 p.m., and I had anxiety wondering how I was going to get through the day. I knew deep down that it did not have to be this hard. I called a sister on the phone, and she talked me through it. I felt supported and I did of course get through the day, everyone made it, and we were fine, but my nervous system, and my being, were exhausted. Knowing I had someone there just to hear me was enough to support me through it.

Having that sister on the phone—a sister who, by the way, is going to medical school and equally has her hands full—was enough to get me through the day. She understood what it means to be overwhelmed, stopped what she was doing, and was there. All I needed was someone to be a witness, to listen, hear me, and be there. She mothered the mother in that moment.

There is so much that a mother handles that only a mother could understand. She becomes so good at caring for the needs of others, and being mindful of the needs of others that sometimes, she forgets how to care for herself. Sometimes, she just doesn't have the energy or the drive. Sometimes, she believes that is just not how it is, and this is her job. Sometimes, there is no one there to help.

This is why we must instill a value system where we care for ourselves and then we will understand how to best care for mothers. If mothers recognize the value in this, I hope that they will ask for the support they need. If families see the value in this, they will support and encourage it. If communities see the value in this, they will create systems to support it.

## CHAPTER 2

# INTRODUCING THE SEVEN SISTERS PROGRAM

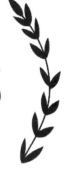

*"Wouldn't it be wonderful if, after your baby was born, someone came to your home and that person understood your needs, and was there to nurture you, answer your questions, prepare nutritious meals for you and your family, and keep your home running smoothly, your way, while you rested and recovered from birth, learned to breastfeed, and got to know your baby?"*

QUOTE INSPIRED BY SUZANNE ARMS

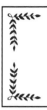
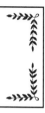

# WHAT IS THE SEVEN SISTERS?

In simpler times, the needs of the birthing family were met naturally by the community. Neighbor women could be called upon day or night to attend a laboring mother. Nearby families cared for her older children and delivered food to nourish her in her recovery. Friends came by to do household chores. And she was most definitely supported and expected to succeed in breastfeeding her infant. Times have changed. Our mothers, sisters, and friends are often not available to help us in our time of need. But the need still remains.

SALLE WEBBER

# THE VISION

The Seven Sisters model was conceived one summer night while trying to understand how I could get the postpartum support I needed. I originally hired a postpartum doula, but she became pregnant and was no longer an option. I had the next 5 months to come up with a different plan. I did not want someone I did not know living with us, nor did I know any other postpartum doulas I resonated with. I knew I required support, but it did not originally enter my mind to ask my friends and family. My dear friend and I were curled upon the couch, ruminating on how to create my new postpartum plan, when she enthusiastically turned to me and said, "What is it you would need?" I told her my concerns, how hard my first postpartum was, and how I was worried that if I did not get proper help, how my health might crash like it did in my first postpartum period. Most of all, I was not looking forward to the feeling of being isolated again. I will never forget her turning to me and saying, "We will do it! Let your girls help you!" I had to let that sit for a moment. I resisted the notion that "your friends would love to support you." It took me time to let that in. We threw some ideas around and came up with the idea of calling upon my friends (who I affectionately refer to as sisters when I refer to the program), and having a sister sign up for a day of the week for 6 weeks: hence The Seven Sisters. We both agreed that this was a perfect plan of action, and I soon began designing my postpartum plan. I wrote up a letter attached to my baby shower invitations that explained that I was asking for help in the postpartum, and why (see Appendix for sample letter). I invited friends to offer the gift of their time instead of baby shower gifts, and only if it came easy to them and they loved the idea, otherwise it would not feel good to them or me.

A funny little synchronicity in the midst of all this. The day after conceiving the idea of the Seven Sisters, I went to the grocery store for my regular shopping, and came out to a rustic old pickup truck parked in front of me with a big sign on the back that said, "SEVEN SISTERS RD" in bold letters on a giant street sign nailed to the truck. I had chills run up my spine. I knew this was something that I was going to design for other mothers and families, and became very excited about how it could take shape.

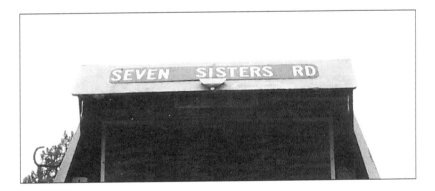

Upon sending out the letter with my baby shower invitations, I promptly received replies from friends with giant YES's attached to them. My friend, who I originally came up with the idea with, has her own restaurant and offered to make my meals in bulk. I told her, "You can't do that!" because

I was so dumbfounded and, as you can see, I had a strong resistance to receiving help. My friend responded enthusiastically with, "Oh yes I can, and I want to! I own a restaurant. This is easy for me!" She went over my postpartum recipe book with me, and even consulted an Ayurvedic doctor to ensure she understood all that was required for the recipes.

I ate postpartum meals that were designed to stimulate digestion, ease constipation, and help nourish the gut. I did this because I had spent the prior years healing leaky gut and knew that during labor digestion slows down, or even shuts down completely as all blood goes to the uterus, and thus digestion is sluggish in the following days. This is just one of the ways I customized my postpartum protocol to suit my personal health picture. The meals my friend made were then offered as a daily special at the restaurant when she prepared them for me. It was incredible.

Other friends enthusiastically responded with what they would love to help with, and my Seven Sisters calendar filled up within a week! I was amazed, touched, relieved, and I felt more supported than I ever have in my life. I distinctly recollect the day I received the e-mail about all my meals being covered from my friend, and the e-mails that followed from my volunteers. At my baby shower, we had a sacred circle, and my mother even came from across the country to be a part of it. She was amazed at the support I had garnered from my community, and I was so thrilled that she could witness what I had manifested for my family and myself. The whole journey was incredible. It truly healed something in me, and has nurtured within me the ability to truly receive help, and to understand how deeply helping another in their postpartum period can influence their entire family.

# THE MODEL

There are many levels to the Seven Sisters Program. In its simplest terms, the Seven Sisters involves a mother calling upon seven (or more) sisters (or brothers) to pick a day each week to support her in her postpartum period for up to 6 weeks or more. She will have your Monday sister, Tuesday sister, etc. Each person will be on call on his/her day to support in whatever way she's (or he's) called upon. It is ideal that there is a point person in place who monitors the team of volunteers, and updates them on the family's present status and needs so that they do not have to think about this during their sacred window of time. With that being said, an integral part of the Seven Sisters is the mama getting very clear on her and her family's needs.

Often I have heard people say that they would "love to help a mother but they do not know how." Or they bring meals, but the directions were not clear for them. The Seven Sisters Program is designed to offer a comprehensive framework for postpartum care. The idea is to make it as easy as possible for the mother and family to receive support, and make it equally as easy and clear to those who would support them, exactly how they can.

I also suggest that the family ask others to only volunteer to do things that they love to do (i.e., if a helper does not love to cook, that is not the offering for them). Helpers can deliver meals, make a meal, do laundry, clean up, bring groceries, hold the baby while mother showers, etc. On many days, I did not have anyone come; they were just on call if I required support. Every Seven Sisters program is customized by the family. How deep and wide it goes is up to each individual family and their needs.

This program is not designed to assess a mama's health status, what herbs she might need, or what meals would most benefit her. However, I do encourage mothers to get clear on their unique needs with qualified care providers to build a customized postpartum protocol. The system is designed to support the mother in customizing the best support for herself and her family based on her individual needs.

# THE IMPORTANCE OF POSTPARTUM PROTOCOL IN THE SEVEN SISTERS PROGRAM

The next step towards setting yourself up with a comprehensive postpartum care plan is constructing what I call "the postpartum protocol." In simple terms, creating the postpartum protocol involves identifying your anticipated personal, familial, and situational requirements in the postpartum period and creating a protocol based on these individual needs. The postpartum protocol is an integral part of the Seven Sisters Program. The more a mother knows herself, her physical, mental, emotional, spiritual needs, as well as the needs of her family, the better she can set up a plan that will support her transition when the little one arrives.

There is so much that a mother takes on that she may not even think about until she's not able to do it. Feeding the baby, feeding the household, sleep schedules, house cleaning, laundry, grocery shopping, taking kids to school, events, and play dates, time to herself (what is that?), doctors' appointments, dentist appointments, school events, and the list goes on! This is why it is so important that a mother and her family get clear on what their immediate needs may be in the postpartum period so they can build their family's postpartum action plan. The clearer a woman and her family are on their postpartum protocol, the clearer their plan can be for those who support them. Another important piece to this protocol is preparing for the what-if's and how a family would like things handled if something unexpected arises: for example, the family stays longer at the hospital than planned, or a home birthing mother ends up transporting. One team, for example, cleaned a mother's house and filled her fridge while she spent an extra day in the hospital. This helped the family immensely.

To prepare my own postpartum protocol, I read many books over the coming months on postpartum care, Ayurvedic postpartum care, as well as books on Ayurvedic cooking for the postpartum, and postpartum herbal medicine. I consulted with my herbalist, Ayurvedic doctor, midwives, and a postpartum doula to create my plan. I had specific meals customized and delivered every few days, and herb mixes for sitz baths ahead of time for easy initiation. I preordered my supplements and made them easy to get to. I knew that my son would need rides to school, so I called upon those who could accommodate this need. I made my grocery lists ahead of time and bought pre-paid debit cards and/or had cash on hand for those running errands. I knew my husband would be overwhelmed with cleaning and laundry, so I asked those who could do that easily to help if it piled up. When it came time to help, I had a detailed e-mail that went out to all the team members about our needs and when meal deliveries were. My point person (which is the person who oversees the Seven Sisters team) coordinated the schedule when there were changes. There were many days when people were on call and I did not require any help because so many of our needs had been met.

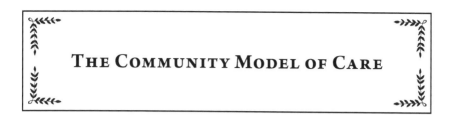

# THE COMMUNITY MODEL OF CARE

The Seven Sisters Model is rooted in community care. I believe that the desire to serve the ones we love is a quality that lives naturally in the heart of us all. However, many of us have become isolated from our families and from the tribal model. We think we have to do it all ourselves, and don't realize that we can ask for help. I have often witnessed that a family will not reach out to their community until they have hit a point where they have nowhere else to turn.

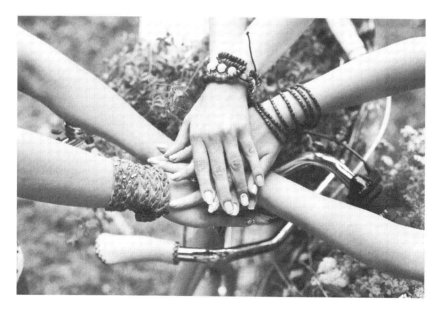

People rally together when there is a natural disaster, death in the family, or illness. It's beautiful when this happens. It's sad that it takes something like that for people to ask for help. People around you likely want to help. It's just that they are often wrapped up in their own lives. They don't know you need help unless you ask. Unfortunately, we have become so accustomed to being isolated, and "doing it all ourselves," that we don't ask for help. Our culture pays little attention to the needs of postpartum mothers and families as evidenced by the fact that we are the only developed nation with no national policy on paid maternity leave.

Something has to change. I believe we can collectively shift this consciousness by helping others see how important it is to nourish a family during this time. Families who receive this level of support are often moved to share it and pass it on in their personal lives and communities. That is the goal of this program: to nourish the model of community care in the hearts and lives of those we serve, with the goal of it reaching out to their communities and our global community. By bringing attention to the need for community care, and recognizing how it affects us all, I hope that we will begin to develop more models to support each other in our communities and beyond.

 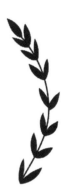

## CHAPTER 3

# SEVEN SISTERS SUPPORT STORIES

*"My message to all mamas who are struggling is this: find your community! Reach out every day. We were not meant to do this alone; we need a village!"*

LORNA DUFOUR
POSTPARTUM MOTHER

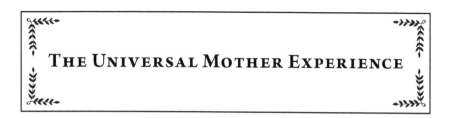

# THE UNIVERSAL MOTHER EXPERIENCE

## Danielle Haines, mother and midwife

I have been working with women becoming mothers for over 10 years before I had my first baby. First, as a doula, and then in the role of midwife. I knew the postpartum could be so difficult. I had seen women struggle more with painful breastfeeding for weeks and weeks, and wonder why she spent so much time prepping for the birth, which was only a day or less. I had thankfully learned of the Seven Sisters Program 6 months before I became pregnant, and it seemed so practical. I loved the idea.

After becoming pregnant, I knew that I would want to utilize the Seven Sisters Model for postpartum support. I was ready for it to be hard and I was ready to ask for the help before I needed it. That was important. To be able to set it up while I was pregnant, know I was going to need it, and know that I might not know how to ask for help when I needed it the most, made it a working system. I also had a meal train set up for me by a friend; we literally had a fresh meal made for us every night for a whole month, and that saved us!

Birth was amazing and intense. It did not surprise me. After attending so many births, and having spent countless hours with women in labor, I had a good sense of how intense it could be. I was surprised at the hormones, emotions, and feelings I felt after my baby arrived. I was so happy. He was so cute. I did it! I gave birth at home! Crazy! My nipples began to crack and bleed. Ouch! I was too tired to sleep. I was too wired from the birth to sleep. My baby was not resting and wanted to nurse on my painful nipples because my milk was not in. Daddy went back to work when we were at 3 days postpartum. I was exhausted.

I had a lot of support, though. I had one of my Seven Sisters coming over that day he went back to work with dinner, thank goodness. One of my greatest friends lived on the same block as me, and she came over more than once that day, and she is a doula, so she knew how to offer me light support! Another friend had popped over for a minute to bring me lunch. I was surrounded by love. But I was so tired, I forgot to sleep. When the buzz of day 3 slowed down, and I was just there with my baby, I started to feel really emotional. I just didn't feel okay to be alone with just my baby. I was worried about a lot of little things.

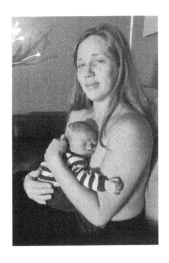

My friend came to visit me and snapped the picture shown that truly captures this moment. It just all felt like a lot: an emotional, open, vulnerable moment. It is awesome to have this image. To see what I was working through. To know most moms will be, or have been, at a breaking point. We need so much more support than what is ever taught to us. We need a village, and yet, they rarely exist. The Seven Sisters program really is a practical way to fill that gap, and I think the program is just scratching the surface right now.

I had so much love and support in my immediate postpartum period that, even though it's a wild adjustment getting into a rhythm with a baby, I had ladies sitting with me through it, for, at the least, every day for the first 6 weeks! The emotional support that was provided with that, and the consistency in support was huge, as well as the practical support: cooking, cleaning, shopping, massage, phone calls, etc. I can look back and remember the crazy, but mostly, it feels like bliss!

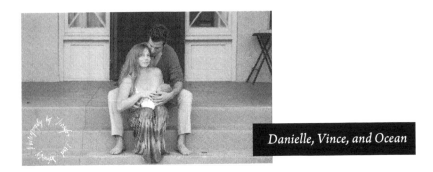

*Danielle, Vince, and Ocean*

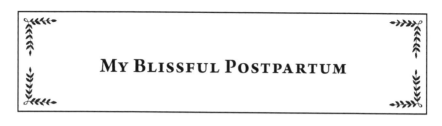

# My Blissful Postpartum

## Lorna Dufour, mother and doula

As I read the postpartum stories of other women, I realize that my story is unique. My immediate postpartum, those first 3 days after giving birth, were the best days of my life! I never left the bed, and being one who loves laziness, it was heaven. I had a challenging, yet triumphant, homebirth, and afterwards, I needed to rest, eat, and rebuild the blood I'd lost. My doula 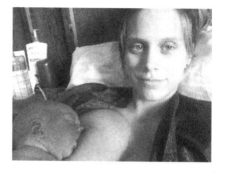 made all that I experienced as blissful as possible. She lived in our home with us for those first few days, came to serve us every day for the following 2 weeks, and was in and out until the end of the 42-day-sacred-window postpartum period. She reached out to my female friends, and set up a Seven Sisters Support network for every day of the week.

When my doula was gone, someone else showed up every day to check in on me. When she was there, someone showed up and offered extra hands. The dirty laundry was taken away and brought back clean. My 7-year-old stepdaughter had play dates. Groceries, diapers, and wipes were delivered to me. Someone held my hand when I needed to walk to the bathroom. Someone held my baby when I needed a shower. Someone was there every day to see me and witness my experience. All of this support made it so that I had zero stress, zero worries, and tons of time for reflection and contemplation.

Mostly I just stared at my newborn in awe. One of my favorite parts of postpartum was being spoon-fed! My hands were tied up in nursing and holding my baby, so getting enough food in me to make breastmilk would have been very difficult on my own. In those first few days, I literally did not lift a finger! I felt like royalty! My doula made healing Ayurvedic postpartum meals, and to this day, those recipes are a favorite in my household! She also made 42 placenta chocolate Buddha molds, one for each day of my sacred window. For me, there was no better way to take my medicine!

My message to all mamas who are struggling is this: find your community! Reach out every day. We were not meant to do this alone. We need a village! The saying goes, "It takes a village to raise a child," but I disagree. It takes a whole, healthy mother to raise a child. It takes a village to support her growth.

## CHAPTER 4

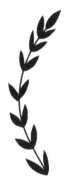

# THE HEART
# OF IT ALL

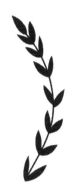

*"After your baby arrives, you yourself may feel like something of a present, albeit clumsy, wrapped in unmatched ribbons and bows, but new. Untried. Untested."*

SALLY PLACKSIN

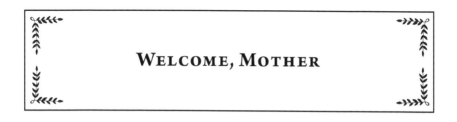
Mothers have been holding the hearts and hands of their children, as well as their communities, since the beginning of time. Becoming a mother is a lifelong journey, one in which you learn about how to nurture not only your child, but also the world around you. You join the community of mothers who are learning, just like you, each step of the way, how to mother, how to love, how to nourish, and hopefully how to care for yourself all the while.

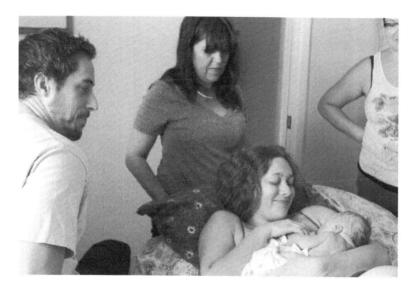

Your child will call forth parts of you that you may have never encountered before. Your heart may be stimulated in places that you did not know exist. The love you have for your child can be a very powerful, healing, transformative force. You will be holding and guiding life, a life that you are now the caretaker of, that depends on you for nourishment, comfort, security, and the list goes on and expands with time. Becoming a mother is a life-enhancing journey. Welcome to that journey, dear mother, and get ready to learn more about yourself than you ever have before.

The initiation into motherhood is different for every mother, but one thing remains the same for all mothers: it is their love for their children. The love you have for your child will inspire you to give everything of yourself. Many mothers do this without realizing what it is costing them. This is part of the initiation—learning how to manage the new demands from having a child.

When your child arrives into your arms, she is adjusting to life outside of the womb, whilst you are adjusting to life with your child now fully immersed into his world outside of your body. All of a sudden, there is a new being in your life, a being that asks much of both you and your partner. This integration process takes time for everyone. Your baby has gone from the cozy space that is your womb to an expansive world with many new sights, sounds, and sensations.

Your body is going through tremendous changes as hormones shift and change, your body prepares to make milk, and your emotions catch up with the experience that is birth. You are learning about your new baby, how to soothe them, and all the intricacies that come with caring for a new one. All the while, your partner is adjusting to this new being in their life. They are learning also how to care for your baby, how to support you as you go through all your shifts and changes, and how to support you in caring for your child.

Your partner is also learning how to balance life outside of the home while also being there for you, however that looks for your family. A lot is going on! You will be walking through many doorways in the early days of your postpartum window. You will feel many waves of emotions as you adapt to this new chapter in your life. All the while, the person you were drifts away into the background, as you emerge into the mother you are becoming.

While all these changes are occurring, I invite you, the mother, to be patient with yourself and your partner. Trust in your instincts and ask for help when you need it. This is a very dramatic, vulnerable time in your life, unique in its presentation in that there are only so many times in your life that you will have the experience of welcoming a new being into your family. Embrace it. Savor it. Allow yourself to be supported by your family, friends, and community.

Many women tell me that they had no idea what would be asked of them in the postpartum window. Many women tell me that they did not know it was going to be so hard. It is hard on many women because they feel isolated and overwhelmed. It does not have to be this way. Your friends and family would love to support you during this time, so let them. Enjoy this sacred window that is your postpartum initiation and, welcome, Mother, to a beautiful journey that awaits you.

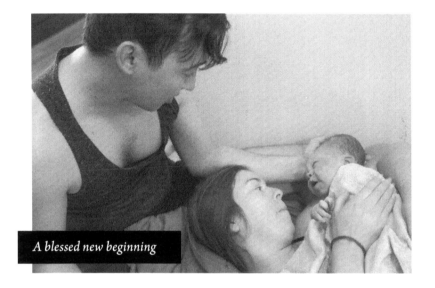

*A blessed new beginning*

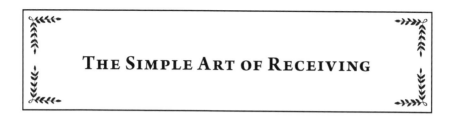

# THE SIMPLE ART OF RECEIVING

To get the help and care we need, we first must be willing to receive. Mothers give everything of themselves. It does not matter if she is a stay-at-home mother, working mother, single mother, or a mix of the above and more. Mothers give everything they can to their children. This goes on for the rest of their lives, and yet, for some reason we do not have a lot of awareness in our culture around the need for postpartum care for mothers of all shapes and sizes.

> I was one of those "I can't" people who wouldn't ask for help. The other side of this is if mothers do not ask for help, then nobody is given the opportunity to help, so it helps both parties. It keeps us all in touch with our needs and abilities and reminds everyone, whether the receiver or the giver, that we are all part of a community.
>
> MOTHER WHO RECEIVED
> THE SEVEN SISTERS MODEL OF CARE

In my experience, mothers resist asking for help. It is the biggest challenge they face in setting up postpartum care. Many women have been raised to believe, and are taught by the lack of postpartum care in our culture, that we have to do it ourselves, and that is just how it is. The model of community care is something that has to be re-initiated in our communities in order to help mothers get the care they need. In many other cultures, this model is inherent, and it is understood that the postpartum window is a vulnerable time for the family, and there are practices in place to support the new mother and family.

Asking for help is an empowering model for the future of our children. It lays the foundation for a stronger sense of social consciousness. Not only that, it is a cycle that keeps on giving. In the heart of one who receives such unconditional help, flowers the seed of passing it on. Every family that I have shared this model with has passed it on in their communities. Every single one. Asking for help during the postpartum window is like asking for helping building a foundation that will support you and your family for many years to come. I encourage people to see it as an investment in a healthy, balanced future.

There are three primary archetypes I have encountered when it comes to resisting this help:

» We have the Superwoman. She who can do it all.

» Fear of Unworthiness. She who does not want to be a burden.

» The Newbie. She who does not even know what help she might need.

# SUPERWOMEN

Superwomen are a creature of our times, and I love them. I believe women can do it all, and I believe they do not have to. The Superwoman is, in fact, super. She can do it all! Many come to her for support, and quite often, she has very little support to turn to because she is so busy being a grounding cord for everyone else. She, too, needs support.

# WOMEN WHO FEEL UNWORTHY

We also have she who feels unworthy. This is a big one, a common one, and a harder one to work with, as these feelings are often buried and run deep. Many women do not feel it is ethical or proper to ask people to stop their day for them. This is so common. After some digging, I often find that underneath this belief is the fear of asking. The fear of being let down.

The fear of no one showing up. You know what? I get it. I get that you do not want to ask others to take time out of their day, and I get that not everyone can. The good news is that people will not volunteer to help unless they can. I have never seen anyone feel forced into helping someone in the post-partum. More importantly, you are worthy, mother, of this care. This is not just for you. This is for the child you are caring for. For your relationship, so you actually have reserves to tend to it.

# THE NEWBIES

Lastly, we have she who does not know what to expect. No one knows how a woman's birth and postpartum journey is going to look. What I do know is that there is a lot more to adjust to when a baby arrives than anyone can prepare you for, and you can prepare yourself to have help set up in the event you need it. And trust me, a little help goes a long way. Know that having extra hands around while you adjust to a new body, a new being in your life and relationship, and a completely new world, is a healthy investment for yourself, your baby, and your family.

> **Dear Mothers-to-be:**
> For people to be able to help you, you have to be open to receiving that help. You are investing in not only yourself but also your entire family.

One common response to the Seven Sisters Model from women is "I cannot ask for that much help." I was one of those women. Even after I had asked for help, and my friend generously offered to make my meals at her restaurant, my response was complete resistance to what I perceived as her giving way too much on my behalf. Her response was priceless, in that she expressed that it would bring her great joy to do so. I received the help, even though it was challenging. I am better for it, and so is my whole family.

The first step to receiving help is being willing to ask for it. Many women resist the community care model because they are afraid to take the first step: to ask for help and, more importantly, to realize they are worthy of that much support. Postpartum care is a preventative measure for isolation, depletion, thyroid imbalances, adrenal fatigue, emotional distress, breast-feeding issues, postpartum depression, and more.

The isolated mindset of "I can't ask for help" fosters more isolation.

# BE CREATIVE AND ADVOCATE FOR YOUR WELLNESS: YOU CAN DO THIS!

Once women are willing to take the first step, which is asking for help, they can get creative in the creation of their plan based on their lifestyle, finances, and community support. Not all people live near friends and family, some will need to call upon volunteers, and this is where the ability to receive is stretched further. Some women will be receiving support from people who they do not even know who will be doing it from the goodness of their hearts. This is a very powerful act, one that can bring a great deal of joy to the giver, and a great deal of healing to the receiver; to know that someone cares, and that they are worth it.

I have been involved in community giving for many, many years. I have delivered meals, clothing, and baby items to people I have never met, and I did it because I loved serving in this way. I did it because I was able to. I did it because I believe in the circle that is community support, and that it will feed itself. More importantly, I do it when I can, and I do not when I cannot. I know my limits. I find we are best served to trust in each other's inner authority and ability to know what we are capable of. People will give if they can, and are inherently beautiful in this way.

Nurturing our community is an act that feeds the hearts of many. People truly desire to serve in this way and seek outlets to do so, as illustrated in community giving when you see fundraisers, and the garnering of support for a family in need. So speaking of community giving, if you are one of the mothers who are put in the position of receiving, please recognize that people will give in this way because they want to. Nothing is making them do it other than their inner initiative and your call for support. They are doing it because they want to. All I ask of those who receive this care is to pass it on. I know you will, because you'll know how amazing it feels to receive it, and your heart will be so full from receiving it, you'll want to pass it on. I trust in this measure.

Say yes to receiving help. Say yes to you. It is possible.

This program is designed to break the old, worn-out paradigm of isolation, which includes the mindset of "I can't." You can! It is possible, and people are deeply nourished by serving the ones they love!

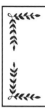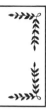

# IN A WORLD OF CHANGE, HEALING HAPPENS HERE

The myths about what we are supposed to feel as new mothers run strong and deep. While joy and elation are surely present after a new baby has entered our lives, it is also within the realm of possibility that other feelings might crop up: neediness, fear, ambivalence, and anger.

SALLY PLACKSIN

Pregnancy itself can be an emotional rollercoaster for many women. Hormones rising and falling, bodily changes, relationship changes, identity shifts, and more. This is a lot to process! The postpartum period is no different. Your body will be going through incredible changes in the coming postpartum days. Your sleep cycles will most certainly change. Your body will be adjusting to life without a baby inside your womb, and your uterus will shrink down to its pre-pregnancy size. Your abdominal wall will stretch and change, and will take time and exercise to return to its original shape. Your body will also be preparing to make milk. Hormones will be dramatically shifting, and your estrogen levels will drop dramatically. You are now a mother, surfing the dynamic waves of new life!

Many feelings arise for new and continuing mothers alike. Something powerful happens to the heart when you experience life that rose from your very cells, and is now in your arms. This goes deep, and there are corners of your heart that are touched that I sincerely feel nothing else can touch.

As a society, many of us were shut down and taught to stuff our feelings. Feelings then become a scary uncharted territory, and many of us have had to learn how to integrate intense emotions without very many support systems set up to support this intensity.

Many women that I have spoken with, report experiencing feelings around their own childhood, and how they were mothered surfacing during their pregnancy and amplifying in the postpartum period. They also may have unresolved fears rise to the surface around their capabilities, especially on the occasion when they are asked to rise to caring for another. The good news is that you are the best mother for your child, and I guarantee you that you will do the best you can for your child.

In my first postpartum, I didn't so much have depression as I did anxiety. The love I had for my son scared me! It brought up deep places in my being, unresolved traumas from my own life journey, as well as my questioning my capabilities to carry out the huge responsibility of caring for another. I had to learn how to feel it. All of it.

Then there comes the lack of sleep, fatigue, adrenal depletion, and, in many women, thyroid imbalances. And here comes a depression/anxiety cocktail for many women.

Prepare to feel deeply when you become a mother. I encourage new mothers to find tools to access their emotions, to explore them, and to be able to sit with fear, anxiety, the what-ifs, and all the emotions that come along with being a new mother. Explore the ebbs and flows of your inner-world and learn how to be with them.

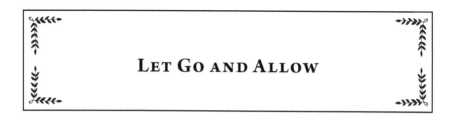

# LET GO AND ALLOW

In order to truly allow others to help us, we must be willing to let go and to be vulnerable. This can different for each woman and family but the theme is the same; a woman must trust in the help of others to let go fully.

"Let me just do it" is a phrase uttered by many mothers, many of which have told me in retrospect that they wished they had let others help them more. There are many reasons why a woman may not receive help, and one of which is an unwillingness to let go of control. Letting go of control means trusting in others to handle it for you. It means letting go of things being done the way you feel they should be done because that's how you would do it. It means trusting that people want to help you, and that they will show up for you. Letting go means trusting. It means letting go of "should." It means recognizing what is most important you and your baby getting this rested time together.

Do not worry about if others put the pans away in a different place in your kitchen than you do, or fold your towels differently. This is a very small window in your life to receive this help. Your pans, your towels, etc. will wait for you. They will wait for you to put them away the way you put them away. Take this time to let others help you with the small tasks. Focus on the big task of resting with your baby, and giving your body the space to heal so you can have reservoirs of energy to draw upon to take up all the tasks you will soon be embarking upon as a busy mother. You will have plenty of time to be busy, to do it all, and be superwoman. You are fully capable of doing every-thing, but you do not have to. Let go and let others help you. The first step to receiving is getting out of the way.

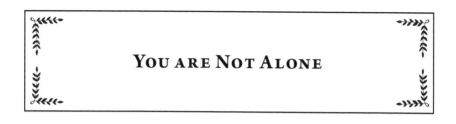

# YOU ARE NOT ALONE

There are women all over the world who spend their days tending to the needs of their flock. Women all over the world who feel the things you do, who go through the challenges you go through, in their own ways. You are not alone in this journey. You are walking in the steps of the ancestors who did this before you, and setting footprints for those who will follow. You, mother, are not alone.

The feeling of isolation is often said to be one of the most challenging aspects of the postpartum period that many mothers face. In my postpartum window, I recall the feeling of being at home alone with my new baby, not knowing if I was doing it "right," not fully knowing who I could call if I needed something, and at times, it was completely overwhelming. New mothers do not have to experience this.

This feeling of isolation can be remedied by being willing to be vulnerable enough to ask for help, and with setting yourself up for proper postpartum care. Just knowing I had friends on call with the birth of my second helped me through this feeling. I no longer felt isolated at all. I knew people were there who understood my needs if I needed to call upon them. Just knowing this eased my worries. Remember, many mothers feel this way. I have often asked my friends, "why do we all sit in our houses alone when we could all come together and be at home with kids together?" I encouraged other mothers to gather at each other's houses, and this is how our gatherings were born. We did not want to sit at home alone, so we did it together. We changed diapers together, fed our babies together, swept each other's homes, watched each other's kids, and cried to each other when we needed to cry. We vented, we laughed, we sat quietly together in peace, and we did it all. We did it because we knew we needed each other.

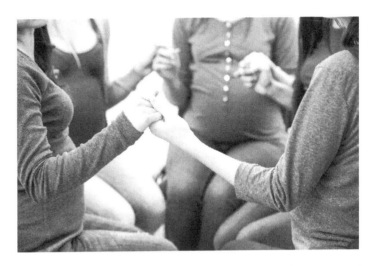

You are not alone in this journey. Gather with other mothers on your lonely days. Reach out to them for community. If you do not have a connection to your mother community, find mother groups, or build your own. You will have the support of your team of course, and the support of the global motherhood community. Call upon them, or make it happen. You are not alone, and all will benefit.

# TIPS TO COMBAT ISOLATION

Seek out motherhood groups before the baby arrives.

Find postpartum support resources, such as La Leche League, baby-wearing and parenting groups, postpartum-care circles, play groups, etc.

Reach out to other mothers. Be willing to be vulnerable and reach out to other mothers for support.

If you feel yourself becoming isolated, call upon a friend to connect.

Build your own Mother's Circle!

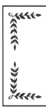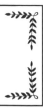

# THE INITIATION INTO MOTHERHOOD

The transition into motherhood, for many women, means being women in the world, to becoming woman at home with child, or woman in the world, who also goes home to care for her child. This does not have to be a first-time mother either. I have seen it with mothers who introduce a second, third, or more children. With a new child comes a shift; a shift everyone has to adapt to, and most importantly, honor.

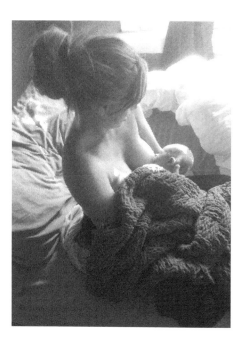

When a woman becomes a mother, she is initiated into the global community of mothers. Many women have been mothers before us, and many will be mothers after us. Many women have walked this path, all across the globe, each in their own unique way. One fact remains the same for all of them: they transform from Maiden to Mother.

When you are woman in the world, you are often caring mostly for your own needs, desires, dreams, visions, goals, and actions in the world. When you become a mother, these desires still run strong in your heart, but this child will take up a great space within you, and will require much of you. I am a firm believer that children do not alter a mother's life so that mothers cannot do all that they want anymore, but in fact, mothers choose to place aside their previous intentions out of a true desire to show up fully for their child and their new life. They are, in fact, a servant to that love. This takes on many forms. For some women, they are stay at home mothers who care for their child all day. For others, they work part-time while coming home to their bundle while someone they trust cares for them. Regardless of how it plays out, they were never a mother until now.

The identity shift that occurs when you become a mother is often deeply confusing for new mothers as they come to understand their new role in life. There is nothing that really prepares a woman for the newness that emerges with your heart walking around outside of your body in the embodiment of your child, to not sleeping like you used to, to not being able to keep the schedules you used to. Your child now often tells you the schedule, and you abide lovingly, a servant to this love. You may have had aspirations that now have been put aside while you choose to mother your child. This is thought to be especially true for those who have unplanned pregnancies and have to integrate the things they thought they were going to be doing. Not only that, but a mother's sense of worth that may have come from accomplishments in the world, and now she's called to find it in this new role. It is not a common theme that people remark on what a wonderful job you have done mothering every day. You do not get a paycheck or a pat on the back, although the rewards most certainly come in different forms; forms that a paycheck or pat on the back could never replace. Yet still, it is an adjustment, and it takes time for new mothers to find their footing.

Feelings of missing the old life often bring up fear, guilt, and shame for mothers. They think they are not supposed to feel these feelings, and many mothers I have cared for have reported to me that they feel bad about these feelings because they should just be happy they have a healthy child. Of course, gratitude for a healthy child is supreme, and also yes, it is significant to honor, let go of, and possibly even grieve for who you were, and welcome the new you that is emerging. It is important to acknowledge the rite of passage you just walked through, and the path you will continue to walk upon as mother. I have met women who have done ceremonies for themselves to create a space to sift through and release the feelings that come up around their new self.

> I thought I could just go back to work a couple of months after my baby. I am an attorney, and I get a lot of satisfaction out of my job, and I realize now that a great deal of my self-confidence was sourced from my accomplishments at work. Once I had my baby girl, I did not want to be away from her at all, and loved staying at home with her. At the same time, I had mixed feelings about returning to work because I felt I had to. Although I loved being with my girl, and I felt less-than because I was at home, I no longer felt like I was accomplishing enough. I tried to return to my busy grind when my baby was 4 months old, only to plummet into exhaustion while trying to manage both my home and work life. My husband and I both decided it was best that I stay home with our ladylove until we were both good and ready, and we are all better for it. This time goes by so fast, and I choose to relish in it. That doesn't mean it still doesn't challenge me from time to time, but it's so worth it!
>
> ANNA, NEW MOTHER

Remember, each phase of motherhood is just that—a phase. I have often joked to new mothers:

> Do not worry, you will sleep again. You will not have mama brain forever, and you will blossom into a brand new and better you! Better yet, you will not regret it! You will probably miss it, and you will long for those sweet, tender, moments at home with your little one.

Trust the process. Welcome to Motherhood, dear mother.

# CREATE YOUR OWN NEW MOTHER CEREMONY

Ceremony, ritual, and prayer, are important components to many of our lives. You can create your own ceremony or ritual around becoming a new mother. This could be integrated into your baby shower or mother blessing, or a separate event.

Invite women in your circle of trust and create a sacred circle together, asking them to hold space for you while you share your anticipation, desires, fears, and personal journey. Invite any mothers in your circle to share with you their wisdom, challenges, and wise counsel. This can be a very powerful ceremony for women becoming mothers, and even those who have multiple children.

## CHAPTER 5

# BUILDING YOUR OWN POSTPARTUM PROTOCOL

*"All women who have made the journey into motherhood know that feeling of being forever changed. After becoming a mother, my emotions reached new depths, and my heart was more open."*

ROBIN LIM

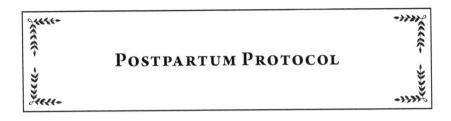

# POSTPARTUM PROTOCOL

A Postpartum Protocol involves creating a supportive postpartum regimen based on your lifestyle, health picture, care choices, sleep choices, breast-feeding/feeding choices, baby-care choices, as well as your designated postpartum care plan and/or team. It involves identifying with your care provider what your health picture is, and what measures you can put in place to support it, your choices in terms of caring for the baby, and keeping a healthy dialogue with your partner to adapt to them together. It also includes being aware of resources in your community that can bring support should you be required to call upon them. The clearer your postpartum protocol picture is, the more people can help support you based on your intended care plan.

The creation of a Postpartum Protocol during the pregnancy is equally as important as the birth plan, for the very reason that you simply cannot fully anticipate all the changes and experiences that come with your post-partum window until you are there. You can, however, create a postpartum protocol to support wellness.

# WHERE DO I START?

If you have never had a baby before, of course, there may be things that you will not comprehend about the postpartum process until you are there. This is natural. Even if you have had a baby, each birth, and baby, is different, and there are things that come up that you will not know about until after the baby arrives. Therefore, the ideal is to set yourself up to have people and tools to call on to support you in a variety of scenarios. The central pieces I have found to a postpartum protocol are the following: healthy, nourishing foods, rest, and support. There are other parts to this puzzle, but those are the top three.

# BODY AWARENESS

Your incredible body that has nourished your baby for all these months has gone through a lot already, even before birth. Birth is a natural process, but still it takes a toll on your body as well as your heart and mind. Even more so if you are not properly nourished, or if a major complication or surgery arises. Nature sets us up for success, and we are best set if we create an environment for healing to easily occur. Being on your feet too much, and putting stress on your body, would not equal creating an environment for healing. Resting, and allowing people to help you while you rest, is a wonderful environment for healing.

# HEALTH PROTOCOL

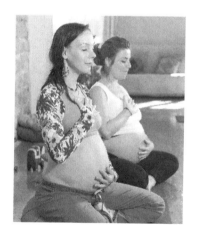

To support your body is to know what your health picture is, and knowing how to nourish your body into balance. If there is a predisposition towards an imbalance, work with your health care provider to get the supports you can to help nurture your body. What I mean by this is if you have a predisposition to a low thyroid and depleted adrenals, like I did, you would call in supports to nourish your thyroid and adrenals make sure to keep an eye on it throughout your pregnancy and beyond. I did this by having my herbalist create a postpartum tea regimen for me that was breastfeeding and baby safe, supportive for the adrenals and thyroid, and overall postpartum health. If you do an herbal-tea protocol, do so under the guidance of a clinically trained herbalist and double-check it with your physician. I strongly advise against making your own herbal protocol, as certain herbs that may be deemed safe for some, may not be ideal for others. In my case, I was referred to lemon balm by a postpartum care provider only to learn from my doctor that it can be a mild thyroid suppressant. Although it is largely safe for others, it was not ideal for me. Thus, it is advised to work with a trained herbalist, and double-check your protocol with your doctor.

# NOURISHMENT

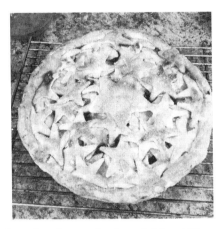

A postnatal woman requires adequate nourishment for the production of milk, energy, and healing. One of the biggest trials for many new mothers I have often found is producing healthy meals while caring for a new baby. Many mothers are also nourishing their families and other children. Thus, food (and hydration) is a very important component to building your Postpartum Protocol.

There are different ways you can set yourself up for adequate nourishment in your postpartum period in the way of food. Getting to know your health picture first, choose foods that are nurturing to your system. I highly recommend eating foods that are easy to digest, as digestion slows during labor, and takes time to get going again. Oily foods, warming foods, soups, dahls, and stews, are all easy to digest while your body gets back in balance. With all of that being said, work with what you have! Eat what feels good and trust your instincts. I highly recommend that mothers create a postpartum menu plan within their protocol to help them get the meals that are best for them.

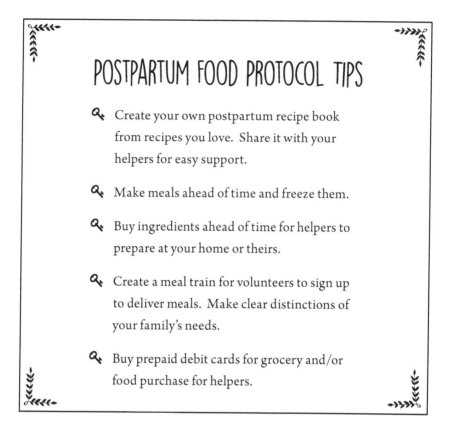

# POSTPARTUM FOOD PROTOCOL TIPS

- Create your own postpartum recipe book from recipes you love. Share it with your helpers for easy support.

- Make meals ahead of time and freeze them.

- Buy ingredients ahead of time for helpers to prepare at your home or theirs.

- Create a meal train for volunteers to sign up to deliver meals. Make clear distinctions of your family's needs.

- Buy prepaid debit cards for grocery and/or food purchase for helpers.

# REST

Set yourself up to get rest whenever possible. All the while, irrespective of how much you nap, your sleep will change with the arrival of a new baby. If you have not been through it, you will not know it until you are there, and I assure you, preparing yourself to get more rest is a huge support tool to nurture wellness, not to mention clarity of mind. It might sound funny that there would be any opportunities for sleep with a new baby, as sleep is often interrupted, but you can create small windows for it. I find the most important step is recognizing how very important it is to sleep when the baby is sleeping if you can.

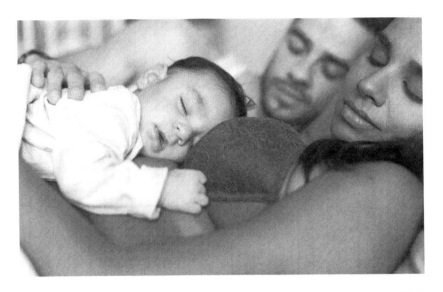

# SIMPLE SLEEP TIPS

- I highly recommend to mothers in the early days after the baby to remove distractions and focus on food and rest.

- Stay in your bedroom with the baby. You will be easily distracted in a central room in the home.

- Keep devices, tablets, and books away from bed as they can easily distract.

- Ask helpers to deliver food and drinks to bedside.

- Keep diapers, wipes, receiving blankets, and immediate baby needs at bedside.

- Have a bed tray you can put on the bed for food and drink.

- Get a changing pad you can have in your bedroom.

# SLEEP WHEN THE BABY IS SLEEPING!

How this plays into your Postpartum Protocol, is setting up your team to support you getting sleep. It is as high a priority as food. Ask people to be with your other children and/or baby if possible so you can sleep. If you feel yourself getting deeply deprived, ask for help. Keep distractions away from your bed, such as tablets, phones, and books that will potentially distract your attention from sleep. Value your sleep time. You will need it.

# SLOW DOWN

**Stay off your feet,** especially for the first few weeks, as much as you can and for as long as you can. Stay off your feet and allow your body to heal. Let people help you by bringing your food to you, your tea to you, holding your baby, putting your dirty dishes away, putting your laundry away, etc. I personally picked my laundry up a few times just out of habit, and was quickly reminded by my partner and/or team members to lay back down. I was just so used to doing it, I naturally gravitated to it. Prepare your team members by letting them know you will be staying off your feet as much as possible, and one of the ways they can support you is by bringing things to you.

**Make it easy for people to find things so you can stay off your feet**. If you are one of those people who just has to do it yourself, it will be very tempting to help people find things in your home if they cannot. This would involve you getting up, and we want you to rest! Make it easy for people to bring things to you by either having a house walk-through before your postpartum window with team members, or even by having labels on important items. Label your cupboards, label which laundry detergent to use, and have your teas out and labeled. Make it easy for people to find things. I know a mother who did this for her postpartum care team, and everyone was grateful for it, including her. Trust me, a nesting mother will have a ball with all of this planning!

**Move slowly.** Have team members in place to support napping. Let this be a priority and recognize the importance of it. Many mothers figure that they will just wing it and figure it out. That is okay, and the learning curve is part of the fun, but having a plan that others understand and know how to support will help you even more.

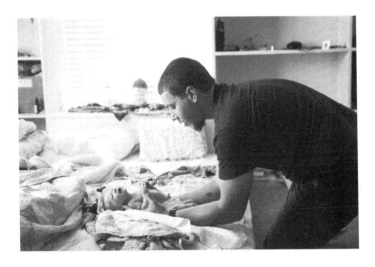

**Let your partner help you!** For some women, this is a challenge, not because she does not trust her partner, but because she feels she has to do it all herself, or only she can soothe her baby, or maybe a little bit of both. It is important and empowering to allow your partner to learn also how to soothe your baby. This is within reason, of course. If it's obvious your baby needs to nurse, or needs mama, then by all means, take care of the baby. However, you'll find that your partner can do a lot more soothing than you'd think, and this is not only good for your partner, but it's good for you and your baby. Many women have told me stories of setting themselves up for burnout by doing everything themselves, or taking a stance of "let me just handle it," and it left them in a position where they had to do it all themselves, and always handle what came up. It was not because their partner did not want to help, but because they set it up this way. Your partner has their own unique set of skills they will bring to the table, and what an incredible, and beautiful journey it is witnessing them bond with the baby.

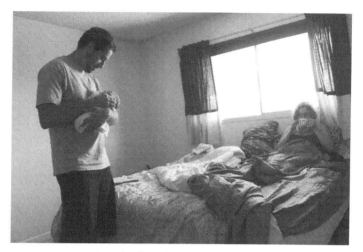

*Papa bonds with baby while mama rests*

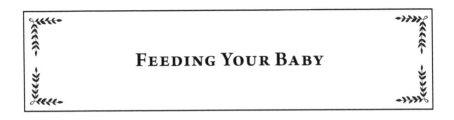

# FEEDING YOUR BABY

*"Being at the breast reminds the baby of being in the womb: there's that familiar heartbeat and soothing voice, as well as the warmth and comfort. And that makes the transition to the outside world a little easier."*

JACK NEWMAN,

*DR. JACK NEWMAN'S GUIDE TO BREASTFEEDING: UPDATED EDITION*

One of the first nutritional choices you will make for your baby is how you feed them. It is an important decision, and whether you choose to breast-feed, bottle-feed, formula-feed, or a mix of the above, there are ways you can prepare yourself for postpartum feeding support. Get clear on how you choose to feed your baby, and familiarize yourself with what your other options are in the event you need to adjust your plan.

# BREASTFEEDING

Breast milk is natural and designed specifically for your baby. It delivers the best nutrition for your baby and provides an ideal mix of proteins, fats, and vitamins. Breast milk is also digested much more easily formula. Breast milk also passes on antibodies that help your baby fight off bacteria and viruses. It is said to lower your baby's risk of allergies and infection. Not to mention, babies who are breastfed exclusively for the first 6 months without any formula have fewer ear infections or respiratory illnesses.

In order that infants and young children grow and develop normally, the World Health Organization (WHO) recommends that infants be exclusively breastfed for the first 6 months of life and then continue to be breastfed, with the addition of complementary foods, for up to 2 years or more.

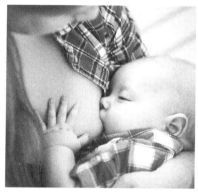

Breastfeeding also promotes bonding between the mother and baby. Breastfeeding is natural, and in the past, most women had no real choice. But not every woman has a smooth breastfeeding journey, and there are many things that can come up that can affect your breastfeeding relationship.

One of my biggest challenges in my first postpartum window was learning how to breastfeed. I did not even think about breastfeeding during my pregnancy, or the fact that it could entail a huge learning curve. For my first week, I experienced excruciatingly painful breastfeeding, with sore, and eventually bleeding nipples, most likely due to improper latch. I never did identify the exact cause, but continued to work on breastfeeding with my baby and toughed it out. Eventually, my nipples healed, and my boy and I found our way. Had I had more support and understanding as to what a latch even was, I probably could have walked through that doorway a bit more gently.

With my second son, my milk was abundant, and he would often get too much milk and then projectile vomit. I had to learn how to position him properly so he would not get too much milk at once, and kept galactagogues (milk-building herbs) out of my tea and diet, as my milk was plentiful. I had plenty of support and understanding on how to handle it the second time around, and it was a much gentler experience, and we worked through it smoothly. I have no doubt any mother will figure it out in the name of feeding her baby, but that does not mean she has to suffer through it.

One of the primary things I have heard from new mothers that challenges them is this unpredictable journey of breastfeeding. To learning how to get a proper latch, discerning if you're making enough milk, keeping proper nutrition in your body to produce milk, overcoming any emotional issues she may have around her not being breastfed, and/or her capability of nourishing another human being. Some women were simply overwhelmed by breastfeeding in public and learning how to do it comfortably. Regardless of the challenge, it is a natural adjustment that comes with motherhood, and every baby brings its own set of learning.

Learn about breastfeeding now, whether you were breastfed, how it went for your mother, and how you feel about nourishing another human being. Also explore your options in the event that a breastfeeding challenge arrives. Know your go-to people and lactation consultants. Talk with other mothers, gather with mothers you know, watch them breastfeed their own babies, and ask questions! There are also the options of bottling your breast milk, or even community milk sharing if breastfeeding becomes an issue for one reason or another. Regardless, you have options, and lots of them. Get to know who your supports are ahead of time.

# MOTHER OF ALL

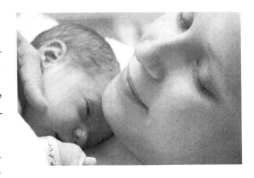

Being the source of nourishment quite literally on every level for another living being, can be quite a weighty responsibility on the heart and mind of new and old mothers. A common concern many new mothers share is the fear that they are not able to nourish their newborn, that they are not making enough milk, or that something is wrong. I remember my own personal journey with this with my first child. I was convinced, even amongst plenty of wet diapers, and healthy well checks, that I was not making enough milk for my son because he nursed every hour, all the time. This is not uncommon, I realize now for a new little person, but as a new mom, I had no reference point, and very little support to turn to.

Somehow in my life, I had never really been around breastfeeding mothers, and I did not know what normal was. With that being said, normal is different for every baby, but this was my son's normal. I was highly emotional for the first week at least, and wondered if I was doing things right because my son was so fussy if he was not at the breast. I also encountered a plethora of emotions around nurturing and being nurtured. I had to iron these feelings out amidst little sleep, little education, and a bouncy-house ride of hormones.

After getting through the first week, finding our rhythm, ordering *Ina May Gaskin's Guide to Breastfeeding*, and slowly having some relief from the hormone ride of despair, I was finding my way. I did some journaling around the emotions that came up, and realized I was working out my own feelings around not being breastfed as a child, around nourishing myself, around nourishing another. I cried a lot and released my fears of not being enough for him, and realized I was made to do this; I could feed my baby, and I trusted in my own instincts and my pediatrician to know if my baby was not being properly fed when, in fact, he was doing just fine. This was just his normal. My little boobie boy.

I came to understand that my biggest challenge, personally, was my fear of not being able to give him what he needed, and I had to look at that and work through it. Once my hormones settled, the pain of sore blistered nipples healed, and I had a book to read through that I very much did cover to cover a few times while a nursing babe rested in my arms. Things eased. I came to embrace my journey and the emotions that came with it. I came to trust in my body. I also came to a place where I began to feel empowered by breastfeeding. How cool it was to be able to feed him from my own body! I traversed many learning curves, such as feeding in public, finding comfort in that journey, and having plenty of tools to help me feel relaxed during the process. Then came weaning, and all the emotions that come with that. Every step of the way, you are learning about yourself as a mother, and again, I encourage you to learn what you can about breastfeeding ahead of time, spend time with other mothers, and embrace the trip that will unfold before you.

# BREASTFEEDING CHALLENGES

There is an array of breastfeeding challenges that can arise, from improper latch, to painful nursing, to trouble with the right hold for your baby, and to trusting you can do it. All the while, there are ample supports to help you on this journey. Your body was made to do this, and yes, sometimes things come up where breastfeeding is challenging, or not possible, but in most cases, there is a solution.

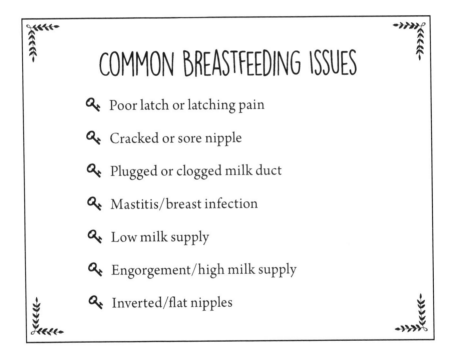

## COMMON BREASTFEEDING ISSUES

- Poor latch or latching pain
- Cracked or sore nipple
- Plugged or clogged milk duct
- Mastitis/breast infection
- Low milk supply
- Engorgement/high milk supply
- Inverted/flat nipples

If you have a breastfeeding issue come up, there are counselors that can support you, as well as mom-to-mom support. Familiarize yourself with your breastfeeding support options. There is International Board of Lactation Consultant Examiners (IBLCE), which are recognized as the gold-standard credential for professionals who work with breastfeeding mothers. There are also peer supporters from La Leche League leaders or WIC breastfeeding peer counselors. There is also the pure wisdom that is mother-to-mother support.

I recommend purchasing a breastfeeding book to help familiarize yourself with potential challenges and to help prepare for your breastfeeding experience. You will find some recommended reads in the resources section in the back of the book.

# BOTTLE-FEEDING BREAST MILK

Many moms want or need to pump their breast milk. To prepare for this adventure, find out how to pump and store breast milk, as well as resources to help solve common breast-pumping issues. Also, discern which bottles and nipples for the bottles you choose to use, as well as review how to prepare your bottles for a feeding and how to introduce your baby to a bottle. Get different kinds of nipples in the event that your baby does not like a certain kind.

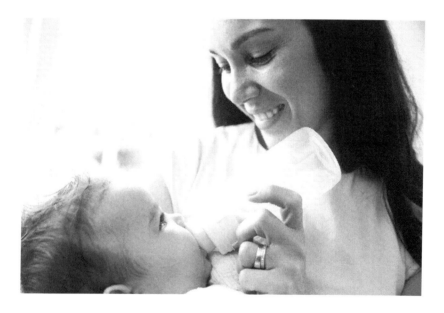

Decide how you choose to warm your bottles, as well as how you will sterilize your bottles. This is a learning curve in and of itself, and you can set yourself up for ample support by talking with other mothers, and deciding what kind of bottle-feeding regimen works for your family. That being said, babies have their own ideas, and that is when already having connections to support networks will help you on your feeding journey. I highly recommend talking with a postpartum-care provider or lactation consultant to learn about proper bottle

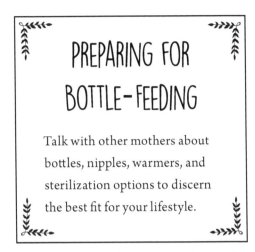

## PREPARING FOR BOTTLE-FEEDING

Talk with other mothers about bottles, nipples, warmers, and sterilization options to discern the best fit for your lifestyle.

holding for both you and your partner before and after your baby's arrival.

Caring for breast milk will become part of your bottle-feeding journey. Some mothers have told me that they wished they had set up a bottle station in their bedroom so they did not have to get up in the middle of the night and walk across their home to the kitchen. This could be accomplished by creating your own bedroom bottle station, complete with your bottle warmer and refrigerator in your room.

# MILK BANKING AND MILK SHARING

In the event that a mother has trouble producing her own breast milk, or has issues with low supply, there is the option of acquiring milk from a milk bank or through a milk-sharing network. According to the World Health Organization, donor breast milk is the best option following one's own milk. Donor milk is only acquired by prescription and the first priority infants are preterm or seriously ill infants.

Where infants are unable to receive all of their requirement for milk directly from their mother's breast, various alternatives are possible. *The Global Strategy for Infant and Young Child Feeding* states that "for those few health situations where infants cannot, or should not, be breastfed, the choice of the best alternative – expressed breast milk from an infant's own mother, breast milk from a healthy wet-nurse or a human-milk bank, or a breast-milk substitute...depends on individual circumstances."

KARLEEN GRIBBLE AND BERNICE HAUSMAN

There is also the option of informal mother-to-mother milk sharing. This is often carried out in close-knit communities amongst mothers who know each other well and have shared lifestyles. It is a beautiful way for mothers to support each other in their communities. It is important, however, to exercise awareness when considering mother-to-mother milk sharing, and have an understanding of concerns and risks when sharing milk.

This is a controversial choice for this reason, and it is important that mothers realize what their options are and how to proceed with milk sharing with the proper education.

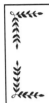
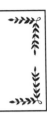

# MORE ON
# COMMUNITY MILK SHARING

### ©Shell Luttrell and Maria Armstrong of Eats on Feets

Community breastmilk sharing works because mothers, fathers, professionals, communities, caring citizens, and people just like you are joining together to help ensure that babies have access to commerce-free breastmilk. Babies need breastmilk to maintain optimum health. Parents and professionals know this! Every day, women from around the world selflessly donate thousands of ounces of breastmilk directly to babies. With Eats on Feets, these donations are commerce-free, just as nature intended, and they are making a huge difference in the lives of babies and their families.

Eats on Feets is proud to be a leading resource for community-based breastmilk sharing.

Human breastmilk is the most appropriate food for human babies. The World Health Organization has even suggested that babies who are fed formula should be considered "at risk." For women who have extra breastmilk, and babies who need breastmilk, milk sharing is the perfect match!

The use of healthy, commerce-free, donor milk is a natural option when a mother cannot provide her own milk to her baby. However, there are risks associated with feeding a baby anything outside of the closed bio-system of mother and child, including breastmilk. It is our mission to provide evidence based information for the safe sharing of human milk.

These four pillars form a foundation from which parents can learn how to safely share breastmilk. The four pillars are not only useful to parents, but also to pediatricians, midwives, and those active in birth and parenting communities.

By understanding these easy-to-implement principles, they too can help babies in their communities by supporting safe breastmilk sharing.

# FOUR PILLARS OF SAFE MILK SHARING

### Informed Choice

Understanding the options, including the risks and benefits, of all infant and child feeding methods.

### Donor Screening

Donor self-exclusion for, or declaration of, medical and social concerns.

### Communication about lifestyle and habits

Screening for HIV I and II, HTLV I and II, HBV, HCV, Syphilis and Rubella.

### Safe handling

Inspecting and keeping skin, hands, and equipment clean.
Properly handling, storing, transporting, and shipping breastmilk.

### Home pasteurization

Heat treating milk to address infectious pathogens.
Informed choice of raw milk when donor criteria is met.

# WHEN MIGHT A BABY NEED DONOR BREASTMILK?

All children have a right to breastmilk. There are many situations wherein a child or baby would need donated breastmilk, including but not limited to death of lactating parent, adoption, foster care, guardian care, low milk production, no milk production, and health of lactating parent. Eats on Feets does not endorse any order of priority for the sharing of breastmilk with babies and young children.

Eats on Feets offers up to date breastmilk-sharing resources for families that desire to make an informed infant feeding choices based on their individual circumstance.

**For information about Safe Milk Sharing, please visit:**

www.eatsonfeetsresources.org

**For information about the Eats on Feets Network, please visit:**

www.eatsonfeets.org

# FORMULA-FEEDING

Health organizations and doctors advocate that breastfeeding is the best thing for your baby. However, breastfeeding is not always possible, and not all families choose donor milk, and in this event, you have the option of formula.

> Keep in mind that formula (like a medication) comes with its own set of risks, and parents need to be aware of these so they can make an informed decision on its use. Parents should look at their individual circumstances and decide whether the benefits of formula use outweigh the risks.
>
> KELLYMOM.COM

There are many different kinds of infant formula on the market, and not all are created equal in terms of their nutrition and digestibility. Following the guidelines as to how formula is to be prepared is equally as important in terms of determining its quality. As with all your postpartum preparations, do your research, talk with other mothers, ask your pediatrician questions, and get to know your options regarding formula if this becomes a route you decide to take or have to take.

When it comes to infant formula, parents need to know a few simple facts.

There are some subtle differences among the major brands of infant formulas, which may affect how your baby tolerates one formula over another. Reading the labels may leave you feeling like you need a PhD in biochemistry to make an intelligent decision. We want to help you with an analysis of the big three nutrients: proteins, fats, and carbohydrates. The vitamins and minerals in all formulas are similar, since these are governed by strict regulations. However, the nutritional fine points of the fats, carbohydrates, and proteins differ from one brand to another, as the marketing departments of each company are very willing to point out, especially to pediatricians.

DR. WILLIAM SEARS

# THE SACRED WINDOW

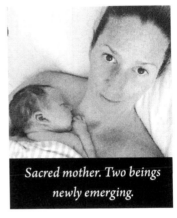

*Sacred mother. Two beings newly emerging.*

I chose a 42-day window for my plan based on what I had read and studied about the belief that the first 42 days postpartum would have an effect on 42 years of a woman's life. In simple terms, it gave me a framework within which to work. I was not attached to exactly 42 days, but I found that it gave me a system and boundary for others, and I felt nurtured by knowing it was there for me. With that being said, I encourage the family to build the sacred window that makes sense for their family and lifestyle.

> According to Ayurveda, the first 42 days influence a woman's health and ability to mother and partner well for the next 42 years. The nature of a mother's unconditional heart makes it easy for her body to either serve to the point of stress, or reset all tissues and systems in the direction of ideal ability to serve, because there is so much reorganizing after birth which must take place anyway.
>
> YSHA OAKES

There are different forms of postnatal confinement in other cultures with different protocol in place. Postpartum Ayurvedic practices were introduced to me by an ayudoula during my first postpartum period. An ayudoula is someone who has been trained in postpartum Ayurvedic practices. This doula was serving a mother in our community as her postpartum doula as well, and would sometimes bring me the overflow of meals, make me a nourishing shake when she stopped by the house, recommend postpartum care practices, and even spoon fed me on a particularly hard day. She was very busy with her client and her other job, but the days that she did stop by made a huge difference, and I took note. I am very grateful to her for exposing me to these valuable postpartum principles.

For my subsequent pregnancy, I purchased books on postpartum Ayurvedic practices and meals from the Sacred Window School of Maternal and Newborn Health to take these practices a bit deeper. I particularly resonated with the beliefs around keeping the mother warm, eating nourishing and warming foods, and staying off my feet in the early days postpartum. I followed this protocol and it made a definite impact. That being said, I adapted Ayurvedic principles with my own instincts and customized my care. I added meat, for example, to a completely vegetarian Ayurvedic menu because I felt better with it in my diet.

The window you designate for your postpartum care is, of course, up to the family. It is ideal to create as much time and space as is possible for the family to integrate together, and for the mother to heal. I urge mothers to let people help as much as they are guided, as all will benefit from it, and you will give it back when you can. There will be postpartum bleeding for up to 6 weeks. Milk will be coming in, and hormones will be rebalancing. Mothers, give yourself time for your body and your being to recalibrate after such a powerful doorway. The whole family will benefit for years to come, and I can share this with great confidence!

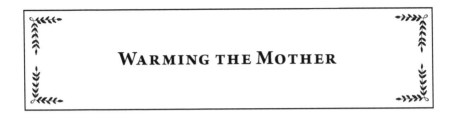

# WARMING THE MOTHER

The practice of warming the new mother is designed to aid in recovery from childbirth and restore energy. This takes different forms in various cultures.

> According to traditional Chinese medicine, heat is highly significant for the woman who has recently given birth. One of the three major factors considered important for the health of postpartum women is "sparing the exterior." According to traditional Chinese herbalist Andy Ellis, this means protecting against wind and avoiding cold drafts. Childbirth is thought to deplete what in Chinese is called *Wei Chi*. The *Wei Chi* is the body's protective immune capacity, found specifically on the surface of the body and in the lungs. Special herbs protect the woman and nourish the *Wei Chi*. The woman is expected to remain indoors for 1 month after birth.
>
> AVIVA JILL ROMM

Keeping the mother warm after birth is said to aid in recovery and speed healing. This is sometimes referred to as "mother roasting" in many natural childbirth and holistic postpartum care circles. In Southeast Asia, mother roasting is a postpartum fire treatment in which a mother lies on a wooden bed above a fire to stay warm. Sometimes they would use heated bricks in place of fire. There are many cultures that employ postpartum practices that involve the use of heat, whether it is laying above fire, covering one's self in warm sand, or the practices in Ayurveda, such as warming foods, belly binding, and warming herbs after birth.

Another way in which we can keep the mother warm, is by feeding her warming foods, wrapping her belly, keeping her head and feet warm, staying out of cold drafts, drinking warm teas, and keeping usually cooler drinks at room temperature.

You can take this as far as you decide, and/or hire a doula that is skilled in these practices. Some of the ways in which I kept myself warm was by always wearing warm socks. I wrapped my belly and my kidneys via a kidney wrap, which involved taking a long wool scarf and wrapping it around my kidneys and tummy, essentially with the intention of keeping my core warm, because a warm core will help warm the entire body. My wrap not only warmed my kidneys, which aided in keeping my body warm, but also supported my tummy as it found its balance again. Postpartum ayudoulas often are skilled in the practice of belly wrapping as well. A few other simple ways that I kept the heat in my body were by drying my hair immediately after a shower. Not going out into the cold without lots of warmth on. Very simple practices that made a world of difference.

Another warming and beneficial postpartum care practice that has gotten more attention as of late is belly binding. This practice serves a much bigger purpose than just keeping the mother warm.

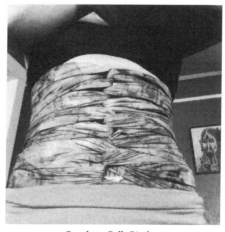

*Bengkung Belly Bind*

Wrapping the belly is an effective and important part of a mama's recovery in the postpartum stage of her journey. It aids the body to shrink and recover in shorter period, normally 6 to 8 weeks. A *Bengkung* belly wrap (pictured) provides a mama's postpartum body with complete support to assist abdominal wall muscle retraction, improve posture, stabilize loosened ligaments, and provide support to the torso while vital organs return to their pre-pregnancy size and position.

VALERIE LYNN

Belly Binding has become popular in postpartum care, and there are many different kinds of belly binds. There is the *Bengkung* belly bind, which is a long cloth that is wrapped by a trained practitioner, as well as abdominal support binders, and post-birth abdominal binders designed for after cesarean sections.

# CESAREAN BINDING TIPS AND TRICKS

If you have a binder available immediately postpartum, you can place a lightly wrapped soft ice pack between your scar and the binder to hold the ice in place. A light wrap is all you need post-cesarean if your abdominals are not separated. If you have determined that you have an abdominal separation of two or more fingertips wide, you will need a more therapeutic/structural binder that can help bring the muscles back together.

Whether you have a scheduled or unplanned cesarean you need to keep the postpartum scene safe, call in your back up, and remember:

» Ask your health care provider for a binder before you leave the hospital—do not assume they will offer one to you.

» Also, ask them what stretches you CAN do within the first 6 weeks to help facilitate recovery.

» Have your insurance pay for the binder or reimburse you if you pay for one out of pocket.

» Share this information with your friends and sisters, so they are prepared.

WENDY FOSTER

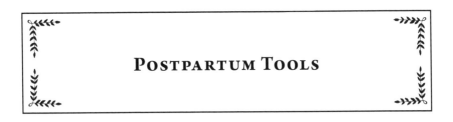

*"Gardeners know that you must nourish the soil if you want healthy plants. You must water the plants adequately, especially when seeds are germinating and sprouting, and they should be planted in a nutrient-rich soil. Why should nutrition matter less in the creation of young humans than it does in young plants? I'm sure that it doesn't."*

INA MAY GASKIN,
*INA MAY'S GUIDE TO CHILDBIRTH*

# POSTPARTUM DIET

Diet plays a huge role in supporting or impeding the body's healing process.

> During labor, the digestion shuts down so that the body can use all its energy to birth. After birth, it is critical for the woman to nourish her fragile and often weak digestion. She does this both for the good of herself and for the good of her new baby, who is to take in her milk; just as the mother's digestion is fragile, so too is the new baby's. Simply eating the right foods at the right time can make the biggest difference in the world.
>
> ROBIN LIM

Ways in which one can support their body is by eating a gentle, anti-inflammatory diet, minimizing foods that are hard to digest, such as nightshades, beans, and dairy, as well as cold foods. Keep the body warm and digestion lubricated and oiled through the use of oiling foods, such as ghee, or healthy omega oils, as well as warm soups. This provides for healing, low inflammation, and ease of bowel movements, which will contribute to a postpartum mother's comfort.

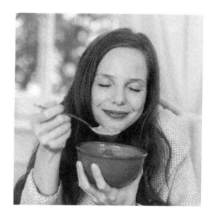

My postpartum meal contained meals of this nature and was based on my personal health picture, which included weakness in my gut. Thus, I paid a lot of attention to eating foods that would nourish my gut. I had discovered in my first postpartum that I had issues with leaky gut and spent the subsequent years eliminating foods and taking actions to heal this. It was of the utmost importance to me that I created a postpartum diet regimen that would support healing of the gut.

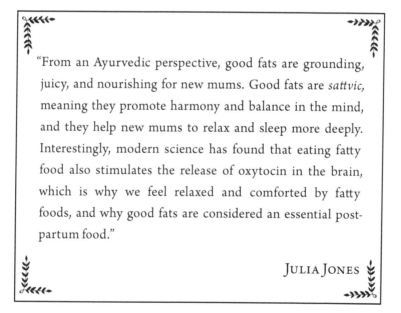

"From an Ayurvedic perspective, good fats are grounding, juicy, and nourishing for new mums. Good fats are *sattvic*, meaning they promote harmony and balance in the mind, and they help new mums to relax and sleep more deeply. Interestingly, modern science has found that eating fatty food also stimulates the release of oxytocin in the brain, which is why we feel relaxed and comforted by fatty foods, and why good fats are considered an essential post-partum food."

JULIA JONES

The postpartum dishes I consumed in my postpartum were warm soups and dahls with plenty of ghee. Nightshades, and dairy other than ghee are very inflammatory foods that irritate my gut, so I made sure to avoid these foods. It is up to you to get clear on what diet is good for you, and do your own research. The Ayurvedic cookbook meals I worked with, for example, were vegetarian, and it became clear to me early on that I needed to integrate meat to feel good. Like everything here, I highly encourage women and their families to base this protocol off what is possible, feels good, their lifestyle calls for, and is easy for their family to carry out. Everything is workable, and that is the beauty of it. Everyone can customize their meal plans based on their family's unique needs.

# POSTPARTUM HERBAL AND MINERAL SUPPORT

Herbs are a gentle way to provide your body with nutritive support, essential minerals, relaxation and calming, warmth, and toning. You can drink herbal teas, have sitz baths, and utilize herbal spritzers, yoni washes, and salves. Work with a skilled and qualified herbalist or physician to build your herbal protocol. Often, midwives, and your health care practitioners who support

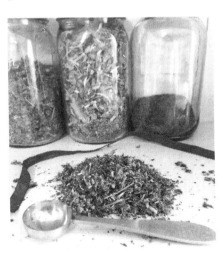

postpartum women, will be able to direct you to a skilled and qualified herbalist.

The herbal protocol I put together with the help of my herbalist and my naturopathic doctor was a hugely effective part of my healing. The protocol we created was based on the understanding that I chose to tone and support my reproductive organs, kidneys, adrenals, gut health, and thyroid. Together, we created an herbal regimen of teas morning and night, not only to support my body in the way of nutrition, but also in the way of warmth. The herbs that I personally worked with as teas were gentle, and safe for my baby to receive through the milk.

# SITZ BATHS

A sitz bath is a warm, waist high bath that cleanses the perineum. Postpartum herbal sitz baths are baths consisting of herbs boiled into a tea, the tea poured into the bath, and then you sit in the bath up to your waist to support in healing any postpartum tears, sutures, or burns. These are incredibly healing and supportive.

You can also get peri bottles (perineal irrigation bottles) to have in all your bathrooms. Fill them with sitz bath tea, and use it as a rinse when you go to the bathroom for any pain or burning upon elimination.

You can usually find peri-bottles for purchase online.

# SUGGESTIONS FOR YOUR POSTPARTUM TOOL KIT

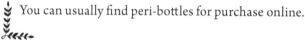

- **Tea press.** Makes for easy tea making, and big cups of tea.

- **Postpartum tea and sitz bath herb regimen** as suggested by qualified practitioner.

- **Thermos.** Great for tea, as well as soup by the mama's bed.

- **Big tea cups** with a nice big handle. Handles are great for mamas who often only have one hand free.

- **Cooler for outside your door.**

- **Do not disturb sign.**

- **Hot water bottle or hot blanket** for belly and/or castor oil packs.

- **Dry erase board** to leave notes outside for team members, if needed.

- **Breakfast tray** for food while in bed.

- **Receiving blankets and/or washcloths to keep close for little messes.**

- **Nursing nightgowns.**

- **Belly wrap,** *Benkung* **Belly Bind and/or kidney wrap** (kidney wraps are easy to make; you can even use a wool scarf).

- **Warm socks.**

- **Nightlight that you love** (For late night nursing when you may need to see what you are doing and it is hard to move around).

- **Bottom balm and nipple cream.**

- **Breast gel soothers to** store in freezer for soothing support when sore.

- **Ice packs** for sore bottoms or breasts.

- **Witch hazel pads** for cleaning the bottom and in the event of hemorrhoids.

- **Perineal cleanse bottles** for easy clean up and soothing any potential ouchy areas (I suggest one to have at each toilet).

- **Boppy**: This is great for nursing the babe, but moreover, sitting on if you have a sore bottom.

- **Small refrigerator** for bedroom for milk storage.

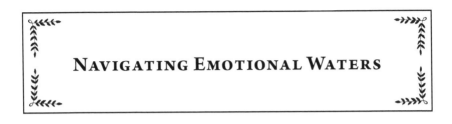
How does one prepare their mind for a baby? This is a good question if you have never had a baby. My answer? Be flexible! What you can know, as I have said already, is that your sleep will most likely be interrupted, your

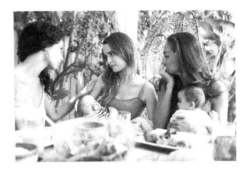

hormones will shift and affect your mood, and your mental well-being is affected by how much sleep, nourishment, and support you are getting.

There are the things that are inevitable, such as the sleep interruption and the hormone dips. However, you can nourish your body to better handle them, as stated below, and develop an emotional care regimen to help support the ebbs and flows of the emotional waves that may very well hit you.

# TOOLS TO HELP YOU NAVIGATE EMOTIONAL WATERS

## Tell your Story

If you would love to share your story with others, please do it. Write about your birth story in your journal for later. Do not worry about punctuation and grammar; just write it out however you love to write things out. Share it with your partner and friends. Let yourself feel the amazing journey you have gone on. If something did not go the way you had hoped, journal about that, feel it, and discuss it with others if you need to. Let yourself be heard and let your emotions be felt. Give them a place to go; a healthy outlet. For me, it was journaling, and for others it may be talking. Give your emotions a proper outlet for release.

**Journal.** Write and release. Anything and everything. Who knows? You may be sharing it later, like I ended up doing.

**Create a "me" time.** This may be 5 minutes, or it may be 30, but try to make time for yourself for meditation, quiet time, or just sitting on the deck with tea. Whatever it is, first recognize that it is a priority for you to have time alone, and set yourself up with your helpers to support you in getting it. You have to value it as a priority and ask for it to happen. Everyone will benefit from it.

**Do not judge your emotions.** You may be emotional, or not emotional at all; you may be overflowing with tears, or none at all. Whatever your emotional state, allow it to do its thing and naturally flow. Do not judge it as wrong or right; it is what it is, and it is your way of moving through this next phase of your journey. A good friend of mine says that you have to feel it to heal it. If something is painful, feel it, and allow it to have its space to move through you. This way, it does not come back on you later or, even worse, get repressed. Not to mention, there are enough people in the world to judge you. Do yourself a favor and don't be one of them. You are doing perfectly. You are the best mother for your child.

**Have a spiritual practice.** If you have a spiritual practice, do not stop doing it once the baby comes. Incorporate it into your "me" time, if you can. Let it be a priority, even if it happens in the shower, or while nursing your babe. This is nurturance for your heart and spirit.

**Call upon a friend who can listen.** If you need a witness, call upon a friend who can listen and bear witness to your story, feelings, fears, or whatever may come up. Sometimes, just being heard is the most healing force of all. This is another way you can ask for help and support yourself. You will find that your friends will be thrilled to care for you in this way. If you do not feel like you have someone in your life to talk to, reach out into your community, and build these networks of support with other mothers before your baby comes. Just talking with other mothers can help you recognize you are not alone and that you are all going through your own respective hills and valleys.

## TOOLS FOR YOUR PARTNER

- Empower your partner to help with care of the baby.

- Share responsibilities and communicate your needs.

- Involve your partner in the creation of your postpartum plan, and help them to understand what you will be going through and how they can support.

- Communicate with your partner what is happening for you and encourage them to do the same.

- Encourage your partner to have self-care measures in place as well.

- Reach out to other partners, and encourage your partner to connect with other parents, for guidance and support.

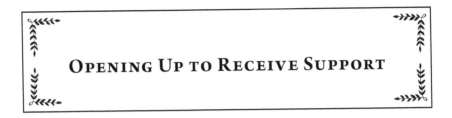

# OPENING UP TO RECEIVE SUPPORT

Many mothers tell me that they do not know how to receive so much support. This is a very common quandary for many women. How do they ask for this help? Women have told me they could not ask for that much help, or they feel like it is too much. I hear you, and I do hope that most women have at least a handful of people who can support them in a time of need such as this. However, you do have to ask.

If there is no one to help, then it is very important to look at your community resources and/or find a way to provide yourself this support with the help of a partner, community systems, etc. to get what you can based on your personal experience. One thing I encourage women to do is ask cherished friends to sign up as a Seven Sister rather than give a baby shower gift. On the other hand, you could ask for help in covering cost for a postpartum doula that could perform the very same tasks as a Seven Sister team.

The other important piece in asking for help is knowing what you require to be supported. This is your job. If you are not sure, then inquire. Ask other moms what they did. Pay attention to your health and diet. Check in with yourself and distinguish what your being is seeking to feel safe, strong, healthy, and alive. If you listen closely to your inner worlds, these answers will reveal themselves to you, but first you must ask yourself. Then you reach out and ask for help. The biggest medicine of the Seven Sisters program is receiving unconditional support. When I received the Seven Sisters support, not only did I feel deeply loved and held by my community, I also realized I deserved to be cared for with the same love and attention that I was giving to my baby. Yes, we must mother our mothers, but in our society, we often need to ask for what we need and direct others as to how to best support us.

Your first step is get clear on what you require. Your second step is asking for help. That is how you ask, you just do it. You deserve that love and care, not just so you will be clear and strong for your child and family, but also because you deserve to be cared for. Period.

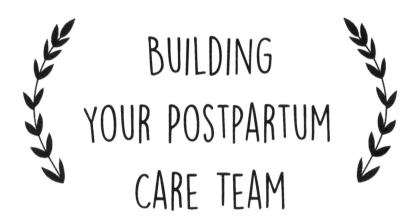

CHAPTER 6

# BUILDING YOUR POSTPARTUM CARE TEAM

*"In those first six weeks a mother should be waited on, served, and nurtured"*

DEBRA PASCALI-BONARO

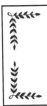
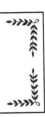

# BUILDING YOUR POSTPARTUM TEAM

The biggest components to receiving the help of a postpartum care team are opening up to receive, identifying your needs, and then asking for help. The next most important component is calling upon a community care team, trusting that your community would love to help you, and allowing yourself to receive such help.

# CALLING UPON YOUR *SEVEN SISTERS*

Who you choose to ask to support you during this time is different for every family. Who you select also revolves around your Postpartum Protocol, and how involved you want your team to be. It also depends heavily upon what is possible for you, situationally. For some people, they center their plan around food delivery, and their Seven Sisters could be a rotating group of people delivering food to their door. For others, it is their closest family and friends coming in and out of the home. It all depends upon how you envision your protocol, your postpartum team, what is supportive for you, as well as what is available to you. Creative thinking and the ability to receive help goes a long way here.

**Assess what you require help with,** and then call upon a team of people you trust. The sacred postpartum is a time of deep vulnerability, and it is important that you ask those who can understand and support your needs at this very special time in you, your baby, and family's life.

# IN THE EVENT YOU FEEL LIKE YOU DO NOT HAVE ANYONE TO ASK

There are cases where women are isolated, their friends and family are across the country, or absolutely overloaded with their own lives, and they do not have anyone to help. In this case, as always, we work with what we have. Up to this point in the text, I hope you have gained a better understanding of what you may need help with, and the importance of slowing down in the postpartum window. This information, in and of itself, is intended to be a stepping stone towards more conscious care in the postpartum window, regardless of how much community care you have. Anything you do to bring consciousness to more postpartum care is a step towards greater wellness.

For women who are having trouble building a postpartum care team, it is important to identify if you are really truly reaching out for help, or if you are only asking a few people out of fear of people not showing up. This is the first piece: Are you really reaching out? If you have reached out, and you find your resources limited at this moment, which it very well can be, I suggest the following alternatives.

## Community Care Teams

Seven Sister Facilitators are trained to organize community care teams in the event that a mother needs help with postpartum care. These teams are made up of both volunteer and paid participants, and are initiated based on the situation and needs. There is also the option of networking with other expectant families, and creating a community care network of your own. This is something I have created in my own community for new mothers in our community, and it works!

**There is also the option of calling upon family and friends who live far away, asking someone to come, stay, and help.** You can cover their airfare and costs and whatever compensation you both decide upon. For some, they prefer this to a doula they do not know. Although doulas are incredible and well skilled, everyone simply has their own vision of how they would like their postpartum window to be. This may only be for a short window of time, depending upon what is possible, but anything helps.

**Look into a postpartum doula for full-time or part-time care.** Postpartum doulas care for mothers as their work. They are well-versed at the things I speak of in this text, and many can customize your care with you. They will adapt to your schedule and needs, and accommodate what is possible. Like with all things, get creative.

## Other Hired Postpartum Care Options

In the event you are still having trouble finding volunteers, it still stands that *any* kind of care will help, and there are many ways you can still set yourself up for greater ease in your postpartum period. I highly recommend hiring postpartum care as part of your postpartum investment in the event that care team is not an easy option for you. This could mean hiring extra childcare, such as a mother's helper, a house cleaner, or chef to help with meals; it all depends on what your priority is. Another option is hiring help to prepare meals ahead of time and freeze them.

Remember, this is an investment into your wellbeing for many years to come. You will be giving every bit of yourself once the baby arrives, so set yourself up to be nourished and nurtured during such a pivotal time. Any help will help!

# TOOLS FOR TEAM BUILDING

## Meal Train

Meal Train is an organized meal delivery that is organized by an interactive online calendar within which friends sign up for a date to deliver a meal after the birth of the baby. It's simple, efficient, and easy to organize.

*Cost: Free at* www.MealTrain.com

## Meal Train Plus

Meal Train Plus is an extension of MealTrain.com, but also makes it possible to organize multiple tasks, such as housework, childcare, multiple meals, and more. This is an even more interactive model that makes it easy to organize volunteers for a variety of tasks.

*Cost: $10 at* https://www.mealtrain.com/learn/mealtrain_plus/

## Seven Sisters Facebook Group

Another excellent tool for team building is building a Seven Sisters Facebook Group for your team to share updates, insights, and to build team morale. I highly suggest building these group weeks before your baby comes to help build connection and communication amongst your team.

*Cost: Free*

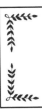
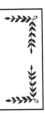

# COMMUNITY GIVING: THE NATURE OF COMMUNITY CARE TEAMS

In my many years of aiming to serve mothers in our community, I have witnessed some of the most beautiful acts of unconditional giving. People come out of the woodwork when there is a call for a family in need. Frequently this group consists of mothers and families who were once on the receiving end of community care. You will be surprised at how many people can come forth during a time of need.

For many, the idea of strangers coming to your home during your post-partum is a bit unnerving. I understand that. Postpartum Community care teams are built amongst the mother and family community, and often consist of mothers, grandmothers, fathers, doulas, and people who love to support those in need. When you call upon a community care team, you call upon your community, which in the case of postpartum care, is often mothers. This could mean making a call out to a motherhood group, creating a Mealtrain.org account with a meal train for a family for people to sign up, or directing your own pre-designed group of volunteers. This is something you can build before your baby comes, by reaching out to friends, family, mothers, and your birthing community.

Community care is built on the understanding that what we give we also receive. It is rooted in the trust that by reaching out you are doing your part in building community, and you will, in turn, give back in the future when a family is in need, and you are able to participate.

Trust in this process, and know that it is a circle that nourishes itself with our careful attention and heartfelt participation.

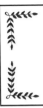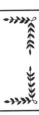

# TIME TO START BUILDING!

*"Good beginnings make a positive difference in the world, so it is worth our while to provide the best possible care for mothers and babies throughout this extraordinarily influential part of life."*

INA MAY GASKIN

Inviting your team members to participate can be carried out in numerous ways. You can write a letter, attach your request for help on a baby shower invitation, ask in person, or however you feel you would love to do it. I attached a letter with my baby shower invitations explaining that I was asking for the gift of time rather than gifts from those who could give it. I went on to express why I was asking, as well as what exactly I was asking for. My team members signed up within 48 hours, and I had a full back-up squad. I was blown away by the generosity of heart that manifested. Just like you create a baby shower registry page, and people sign up and purchase what they'd love to get for you, you are asking for the gift of time, and specific skills. The only difference is it involves time, and not goods; the initiative to receive help from those who love you, and asking for it, is the same.

When you ask for help, it helps to include the following:

- ✎ Asking for the gift of time.

- ✎ Specifying exactly what you are asking for help with and how it would work.

- ✎ Expressing why you are asking for this help and how it will support your family.

If people who do not live close to you want to donate to your Postpartum Care program, they can support by either giving gift cards that you can give to support people when they run errands for you, or they can support by buying items on your postpartum care list. Another way they could support is putting money towards you receiving postpartum doula care if this is the route you choose to take. If you decide to go with a doula, you can have her co-design your plan based on how she works, so rather than a team, it would be your doula carrying out the intention.

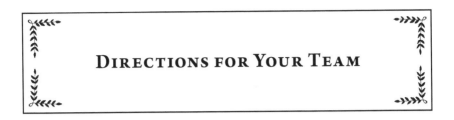

# YOUR POINT PERSON

Once you have a team of volunteers, elect a point person who will guide the entire team. If possible, find someone who knows you and your family well. An ideal point person is also organized and a good communicator. Another piece to consider is making sure the point person is not overstretched also. I say this because, often, other mothers offer to take on this role and they too have to make sure they can truly do this in a balanced way whilst managing their own family. The idea is for it to be sustainable for all involved.

I affectionately call the point person "the gatekeeper," in that they will be fielding all the calls and questions, as well as giving information to volunteers as to what you may be needing on a given day. Many people tell me their partner can be their point person, but I advise against this so that the partner can direct their energy towards the mother, baby, and family, and not fielding calls and questions. There will be some degree of that, but it is ideal for the partner not to be the primary point person.

Preferably, the point person is just that, the person who organizes the team, calls, and questions as stated above. However, a point person can also volunteer one or more days a week, or just be in charge of team directing. That is up to you and your point person.

In my case, my point person was myself. I did not think to have someone else do it, as I was the one who created my plan, so I directed it. I first sent out an initial call for help with my baby shower invitation, asking for the gift of time. I had a quick response from dear friends who offered to volunteer, upon which we went over what we required help with, and specified who could help with what, and when. Each friend had a day of the week that they were on call. Some friends just did meal delivery, sometimes for a few days a week. When the baby came, my husband texted my friend, who was coordinating the meals, and the meals began coming. Upon day 3, I emailed everyone and let them know what I required help with, and that I would text people on their day if I needed help. They were on call during their day for their allotted time (e.g., one woman would always come on Tuesdays at 11, and I had to text her if I did not require help that day).

My primary friend, who organized my meals, would also check in with my husband or me, and would direct people to drop off food. I also had a friend who came on Wednesdays to play with my son, and another who would come and make food once a week at my home. I would receive a gallon of food (usually a soup) from the restaurant at a time, so I often would direct other providers to not come for a few days, as I was well-taken care of with food and was not concerned about laundry/house cleaning upon which volunteers, being the lovely women that they are, would often do it anyway if they were at the home. I learned how to receive it, but not without a little resistance. In the end, when I look back on it, I am deeply moved by how loved I was by my community, and the unconditional giving that came through these women. My family will forever be better for it.

# ONCE YOU HAVE YOUR POINT PERSON IDENTIFIED, CALL A TEAM MEETING.

At your team meeting, you will go over your plan with your team, explore questions, concerns, insights, and prepare a plan for the delivery of your Seven Sisters Plan.

You will also make sure all your team members know their way around your house, know where to find items that you will require during your time, and ask any questions in this regard.

One mother receiving postpartum care labeled everything. She labeled her kitchen cupboards, her laundry soap, and made lists for her caretakers. Label makers come cheap, and they do make adhesive labels that do not strip paint off cabinets, if this is something you wanted to do.

Distribute a copy of the plan to all of your team members with everyone's phone numbers and directions. There are sample sheets at the end of the manual to guide how to make these. They are quite simple. Make sure all team members understand how you would like the plan to be carried out, and that the point person knows how to guide the team, and that team members know they are the person to go to with questions once the baby comes.

Have back up people in the event someone cannot participate on a given day.

# HAVE A BACK—UP PLAN

In the event of an extended hospital stay or unexpected transfer, have someone prepare the home for the mama and baby's arrival.

Have food ready at the home, and check hospital policies and see if food can be delivered there.

Know your postpartum care providers ahead of time, such as Breastfeeding counselors, body workers, postpartum care providers, back up childcare, etc.

Make sure your point person has access to back-up plan details as well as contact info for postpartum care providers in the event that they need to be contacted.

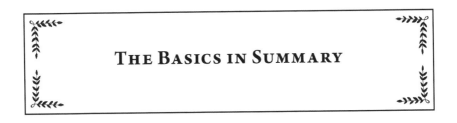

# THE BASICS IN SUMMARY

## Get clear, deep within yourself, on what you envision as a nurturing, supportive, healthy postpartum period.

Get clear with your care givers and health care providers about what your body is requiring to maintain health through pregnancy and beyond. If you have health conditions that are a concern to you, seek out a health practitioner of your personal preference to help you get clear on your personal plan. It is important to team up with someone who you resonate with and who understands your needs. Once you have a clear picture of what you are requiring on a physical level, you can seek out and set up supportive measures in the way of diet, herbs, and supplements/medications if required, in your immediate postpartum.

## Identify your care team.

Pick women (or men) who you feel safe with, ones who understand who you are and how to support you. If you do not feel like you have people like this in your life, then seek out those you trust the most, and *teach* them how to best support you. It is a challenging piece for many women to ask for what they need, but if you choose to receive help, you often have to ask others for exactly what you need so they can best help you. It is one of the gifts of the Seven Sisters to learn that you are worthy of receiving such love. Yes, you are, mother. Yes, you are!

## Clarify your familial and household needs.

If you do not know what these could possibly be, ask other mothers, and inquire with women in your community. It is valuable to not just ask for meals, because when a child comes, it is ideal that you are able to lay in with them, if possible, and let others handle *all* other tasks. This means house-keeping, grocery shopping, putting out the garbage, tending to other kids, etc. In my case, I have a toddler and horses. Thus, I required people to help get my toddler to preschool, feed my horses, and muck my pens, not to mention food and light housekeeping. I did not choose for all of this to fall upon my husband's shoulders, and made a point to arrange a team to help me in this way. I am so glad that I did it because it would have been a huge weight for all of us. I had friends helping with my kids, and it flowed beau-tifully. It was hard for me to sit back and let everyone handle it, but I knew deep down that this was the best thing I could possibly do.

## The clearer you are, the better your team can support you.

This is very important. The more organized and clear you are, the easier things will flow, not only for your team, but also for you. If your team has to keep checking in with you because they do not know what to do, this inter-rupts your rest, and your ability to just sit back. There are many ways you can offer this clarity to your team.

# YOUR NEXT STEPS

## Appoint your point person.

This person is someone who is grounded, organized, and able to commit to your designated postpartum care window of being the person who keeps your team informed. This person will contact your team, and initiate them when the baby comes. They will update them on your needs and desires. They will be the contact person so you don't have to do any of it.

In the event that you are the point person, set up your means of commu-nication in a way that makes it easy on you. Make sure everyone is clear ahead of time on how to proceed once the baby arrives.

**Have a meeting with your team** and point person to show them around your house. Educate your team members about the intricacies of your house so, once again, you do not have to be interrupted when you are in bed. Show them how to work the dishwasher and washing machine. Stock up on the detergents you love and make them readily available. Show them how to move around your kitchen. If they are watching your kids, have them have a playdate or two, or three before the baby comes. Prepare everyone so the transition is as smooth as possible for (the unknown is always a factor and we recognize this).

This, again, requires planning, and a willingness to ask for help. If people have offered to support you in this way, they want to support you. So let them. Make it easy on them and you. The more clarity and communication there is, the easier it is for everyone.

**Have a backup plan** if something comes up that you did not plan for. Much like we have the birth plan, this is your postpartum plan.

Setting up your Seven Sisters team is a gift not only to yourself, but to your future health and your family's harmony. When our mothers' cups are full, their entire family benefits from their harmonious and healthy embodied presence.

# THE BASICS OF BUILDING YOUR SEVEN SISTERS CIRCLE

1. Be willing to ask for, and *receive* help.

2. Get clear on you and your family's needs: your physical, mental, emotional, spiritual, and situational needs.

3. Design your postpartum protocol and purchase (or ask for items as gifts) to support it.

4. Call upon your friends, family, and community to set up a team.

5. Identify a point person for your team.

6. Have a team meeting and go over your plan with your team. Give your team a tour of your house, and make sure they know where everything is for the postpartum plan.

7. Have back-up team members, if possible.

8. Have a back-up plan, and make sure members know how to carry it out.

9. Sit back and receive loving support from your team when your baby arrives.

10. Pay it forward, and offer support to family, friends, and community when you are able.

11. Share with others how to support mothers in their postpartum, like you were supported.

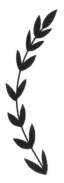

CHAPTER 7

# WORKSHEETS
# AND
# EXERCISES

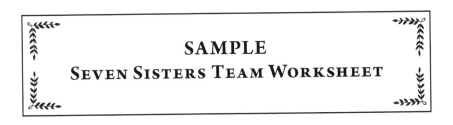

# SAMPLE
## SEVEN SISTERS TEAM WORKSHEET

This is handed out to all team members at your team meeting, and you would go over it to make sure everyone understands it.

| TEAM MEMBERS | | PHONE NUMBERS |
|---|---|---|
| **Monday** | Dinah | 555-1234 |
| **Tuesday** | Mary | 555-3214 |
| **Wednesday** | Henry | 555-7894 |
| **Thursday** | Lilah | 555-6547 |
| **Friday** | Jenny | 555-8521 |
| **Saturday** | Kelly | 555-0321 |
| **Sunday** | Lorenzo | 555-7412 |
| **Back Up** | Michaela | 555-6321 |
| | Olive | 555-8564 |
| | Noah | 555-4569 |
| | Rose | 555-4567 |

All are on call to fill in any day with 24-hour notice.

**Point Person: Teresa**      **555-2589**

Teresa will text when plan is activated.

# PLAN

**Meal Delivery:** Lunch and Dinner. Please text before drop-off to confirm. Cooler out front if sign is on door. Text before delivery. If there is no sign on door, you are welcome to knock, or put in fridge if I am sleeping.

**Meal restrictions:** No gluten or dairy. Be mindful of nightshades, beans/legumes, heavy foods during first week.

**Recycling:** Recycling will be out front for delivery when needed.

**Grocery shopping:** Grocery list with cash will be provided on Monday and Friday. Please put in fridge. You are welcome to pick up cash/list on Sunday and Thursday to carry out shopping following day. Will be left in envelope out front with "Groceries" written on it.

**Help with Baby:** Mom will text you if it is your day, and she needs help, to see if you are available.

**Be Mindful:** It will be exciting to see mom and baby. Family will be lying in. A Do Not Disturb sign will be on door when they are resting. Please check sign on front door to see if they are up to visiting.

**Lastly:** If you have ANY questions, contact our point person Teresa at 555-2589

## THANK YOU!

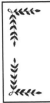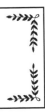

# SEVEN SISTERS
## TEAM WORKSHEET TEMPLATE

(This would be handed out to all team members at your team meeting and you would go over it to make sure everyone understands it).

| TEAM MEMBERS | PHONE NUMBERS |
|---|---|
| **Monday** _____ | _____ |
| **Tuesday** _____ | _____ |
| **Wednesday** _____ | _____ |
| **Thursday** _____ | _____ |
| **Friday** _____ | _____ |
| **Saturday** _____ | _____ |
| **Sunday** _____ | _____ |
| **Back Up** _____ | _____ |
| _____ | _____ |
| _____ | _____ |

*(All are on call to fill in any day with 24-hour notice.)*

**Point Person:** _____

# PLAN

**Meal Delivery:**

_____

_____

_____

_____

**Meal restrictions:**

_____

_____

_____

_____

**Other:**

_____

_____

_____

_____

_____

**Lastly:** If you have ANY questions, contact our point person

## THANK YOU!

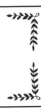

# SAMPLE INVITATION

Dear Friend,

As we prepare for the arrival of our wee one, we are inviting our friends to give the gift of time rather than baby shower gifts. The postpartum period is a very vulnerable time for the family, and we have chosen to set up a team as a nurturing safety net to help get the care we require in the postpartum period. We are asking you to participate if you feel called and it is easy for you. We encourage you to only volunteer for tasks that you love to do. We are setting up a postpartum care team based on the Seven Sisters Model of Community Care. This model is designed for up to 6 weeks, upon which we have a person sign up for one day a week, each week, to volunteer their time for a personalized designated time slot.

We also require a point person to help direct the team, someone who loves the idea of organizing the group, making the calls when the baby arrives, and fielding any questions. Please see subsequent note with the tasks we are asking for support with.

The day you choose would be your on-call day. Or you can slot out a time that works for you, and/or share the day with another.

Please let us know if you are interested in participating in this way and, again, we are asking for this in lieu of gifts, and only from those who are easily able to contribute in this way.

Thank you for being in our lives and being a part of this special time!

Signed,

_____

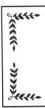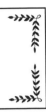

# SAMPLE SEVEN SISTERS
# ADDENDUM TO LETTER

Rather than gifts at our baby shower, we are asking for the gift of your time, but only if it is easy for you, you love the idea, and it comes naturally. We ask that you only volunteer for what you love to do, and please recognize this is not obligatory in any way, as we know life is busy!

On the next page are our *Seven Sister Days* and tasks we are asking for help with. Please check off any tasks you love, and day or days that are possible. We will formulate a set schedule at team meeting where you will be assigned one day.

The time you put in on that day is up to you.

We will be having a point person, or persons, who will be directing the entire team in the way of organizing the schedule, contacting everyone when the baby arrives, and fielding questions if they come up once the baby arrives. Would you like to be a point person? _____

This schedule will be activated as soon as the baby arrives. We will also have a meal train running, which the point person will activate once the baby arrives to initiate the delivery of meals. If you'd love to help via the meal train, you can find that link here: www.mealtrain.org

Thank you for being a part of our postpartum care team. The postpartum is one of the most vulnerable times in a woman and family's life. Seeing as the model of "the village" is lacking in our present day society, we are creating our village, in the name of giving our baby and family as much support as we can to make this transition gentler.

We appreciate you, and thank you!

If you have any questions, about this program, you can check it out at www.sevensisterspostpartum.com, or we welcome your questions, as we will open time for discussion about this if any questions arise, at our baby shower.

| TASKS | MON | TUES | WED | THUR | FRI | SAT | SUN |
|---|---|---|---|---|---|---|---|
| Childcare/Taking Toddler to School | | | | | | | |
| Meal Preparation | | | | | | | |
| Errands/Grocery Shopping/Recycling | | | | | | | |
| Laundry | | | | | | | |
| Light Housekeeping | | | | | | | |
| Baby Watching/Wearing | | | | | | | |
| Miscellaneous | | | | | | | |

# MAMA MEDITATION

Being able to be with your emotions, which are often an ever-changing river ride during the postpartum, is a medicine that can bring great comfort to both mother, child, and the entire family unit. I encourage mothers to become familiar with what I call their inner world (their emotions, feelings, beliefs), and develop a compassionate disposition towards their fears, challenges, and growth opportunities. One way a mother can do this is with a tool I call the Mama Meditation. This meditation is simple is a tool for self-inquiry to get an understanding around what emotions are coming up so you can discern how to navigate them and work with them consciously. This is not designed to be a solution or a way to fix what you are feeling, but to identify it. Feelings are first meant to be felt, and what follows is different for everyone. Sometimes, it's just a feeling that needs to be witnessed, and that is all that needs to occur. Other times, the feeling requires first to be felt, witnessed, and then action is required to bring resolve. I find that in the postpartum window, with so many feelings rising and falling in the open heart of the mother, it is simply about being willing to feel, to surrender to the wave and let your boat coast the changing tides. For the Mama Meditation, all that is required is a quiet space (nursing a babe is even quite a wonderful place to do this), and a willingness to listen. A journal is recommended, but not required.

# MAMA MEDITATION

Q. Sit or lay quietly (sitting ideal) and close your eyes.

Q. Pay attention to your breathing. Breathe in deeply, all the way into your belly, and exhale slowly. Keep consciously breathing until you feel a quiet calm come over you.

Q. Now direct your attention to what emotions are rising and falling. Watch them like clouds passing by in a cloudy sky.

Q. If you are curious about a feeling that is arising, ask: "What do you need to show me?"

Q. The answer may be more feeling. It may be images. The intention is to bear witness to your emotions, and allow them to be felt, and to reveal anything they have to share.

Q. If it feels relevant, write down what comes up. Be gentle with your feelings. Do not try to solve anything. Just bear witness to it.

Q. I find it helps to sleep on anything that comes up that you feel needs to be addressed. Take time to let it settle, and then revisit it.

# ABOUT THE AUTHOR

Michelle Peterson is the founder of The Seven Sisters Postpartum Care Program. As a mother of two sons, and a wife deeply involved with her community, Michelle has focused on the path of motherhood and community consciousness around the need for natural childbirth, postpartum care, and the spiritual, emotional, and physical welfare of families as the backbone of our collective well-being. Michelle teaches the Seven Sisters Model to pregnant women and new mothers and their families. She also offers a series of classes to people who would love to become facilitators offering the Seven Sisters model to mothers and families in their community.

**You can learn more about the
Seven Sisters Program and Upcoming Trainings at
www.SevenSistersPostpartum.com**

# Resources

## Ayurvedic Postpartum Care

Sacred Window School for Maternal and Newborn Health: www.sacredwindow.com

The Mommy Plan by Valerie Lynn

## Belly Binding

The Mommy Wrap: https://themommyplan.com/recoveryproducts/

## Breastfeeding

### Books

The Womanly Art of Breastfeeding by Diane Wiessinger, Diana West, and
    Teresa Pitman

The Family Nutrition Book: Everything You Need to Know About Feeding Your
    Children- From Birth through Adolescence by William Sears, MD and
    Martha Sears, RN.

Ina May's Guide to Breastfeeding by Ina May Gaskin

Dr. Jack Newman's Guide to Breastfeeding by Jack Newman, MD

Breastfeeding Made Simple: Seven Natural Laws for Nursing Mothers by
    Nancy Mohrbacher, IBCLC and Kathleen Kendall-Tackett, PhD, IBCLC

### Websites

Milk Sharing: www.eatsonfeets.org

Kelly Mom: www.KellyMom.org

Dr. Jack Newman: http://www.nbci.ca

Breastfeeding Online: http://www.breastfeedingonline.com/newman.shtml

Lactmed-Drugs and Lactation Database: https://toxnet.nlm.nih.gov/newtoxnet/
    lactmed.htm

Breastfeeding Made Simple: www.breastfeedingmadesimple.com

## Herbs

### Books
*Healing Wise* by Susun Weed

Aviva Romm

### Websites
Earth Mama Angel Baby www.earthmamaangelbaby.com

## Postpartum Recipe Books
*First Forty Days* by Heng Ou

## Postpartum Care
*After The Baby's Birth* by Robin Lim

*Natural Health After Birth* by Aviva Romm

## Baby Care Products
Ergo www.ergo.com

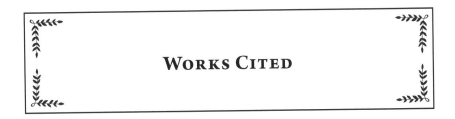

# WORKS CITED

## CHAPTER 1
### The Importance of Postpartum Care

Arms, Suzanne. "Suzanne Arms." *www.birthingthefuture.org*. Suzanne Arms, n.d. Web. <http://birthingthefuture.org/>.

Kim-Godwin, Yeoun Soo. "Postpartum Beliefs and Practices Among Non-Western Cultures." MCN, The American Journal of Maternal/Child Nursing 28.2 (2003): 74-78. Web. 06 Apr. 2016. <http://www.birthways. com/girlnet_docs/Postpartum_Beliefs.pdf>.

Kendall-Tackett, Kathleen. "How Other Cultures Prevent Postpartum Depression Social Structures That Protect New Mothers' Mental Health." *UppityScienceChick.com*. Kathleen Kendall-Tackett, n.d. Web. <http://www. uppitysciencechick.com/how_other_cultures.pdf>.

Lim, Robin. *After the Baby's Birth-- A Woman's Way to Wellness: A Complete Guide For Postpartum Women*. Berkeley, CA: Celestial Arts, 1991. Print.

Oakes, Ysha. *Touching Heaven, Tonic Postpartum Care and Recipes with Ayurveda*. 3rd ed. Alburquerque, NM: Ysha Oakes, 2012. Print.

Panettiere as quoted by Johnson, Zach. "Hayden Panettiere Opens Up About Her Postpartum Depression: "Women Need to Know That They're Not Alone"." E! Online. N.p., n.d. Web. 05 May 2016. <http://www.eonline. com/news/700967/hayden-panettiere-opens-up-about-her-postpartum-depression-women-need-to-know-that-they-re-not-alone>.

## CHAPTER 2
### Introducing the Seven Sisters Program

Arms, Suzanne. "Suzanne Arms." *www.birthingthefuture.org*. Suzanne Arms, n.d. Web. <http://birthingthefuture.org/>.

Webber, Salle. *The Gentle Art of Newborn Family Care: A Guide for Postpartum Doulas and Caregivers.* Amarillo: Praeclarus, 2012. Print.

## CHAPTER 4
### The Heart of it All

Placksin, Sally. *Mothering the New Mother: Women's Feelings and Needs after Childbirth: A Support and Resource Guide.* New York: Newmarket, 2000. Print.

## CHAPTER 5
### Building Your Own Postpartum Protocol

"Choosing Formula." Ask Dr Sears The Trusted Resource for Parents. www.AskDrSears.com, 23 Aug. 2013. Web. 02 July 2016. <http://www.askdrsears.com/topics/feeding-eating/bottle-feeding/choosing-formula>

Foster, Wendy. "Cesarean Survival Essentials: Postpartum Binding." International Cesarean Awareness Network. Icanonline.org, 9 Dec. 2015. Web. 07 July 2016. <http://www.ican-online.org/blog/2015/12/cesarean-survival-essentials-postpartum-binding

Gaskin, Ina May. *Ina May's Guide to Childbirth.* New York: Bantam, 2003. Print.

Gribble, Karleen D., and Bernice L. Hausman. "Milk Sharing and Formula Feeding: Infant Feeding Risks in Comparative Perspective?" The Australasian Medical Journal. Australasian Medical Journal, 31 May 2012. Web. 03 July 2016. <http://www.ncbi.nlm.nih.gov/pmc/articles/PMC3395287/>.

Jones, Julia. "Why Ghee Is the Perfect Postpartum Food." Newborn Mothers. Julia Jones, 28 Mar. 2016. Web. 3 July 2016.

KellyMom.com "What Should I Know about Infant Formula? • KellyMom.com." KellyMomcom. N.p., 02 Aug. 2011. Web. 02 July 2016. <http://kellymom.com/nutrition/milk/infant-formula/>.

Lim, Robin. *After the Baby's Birth: A Woman's Way to Wellness: A Complete Guide For Postpartum Women.* Berkeley, CA: Celestial Arts, 1991. Print.

Lim, Robin. "Postpartum: Rebirth of the Woman by Robin Lim." *Postpartum: Rebirth of the Woman.* N.p., 2003. Web. 07 July 2016. <https://www.midwiferytoday.com/articles/postpartum_rebirth.asp>.

Lynn, Valerie. *The Mommy Plan: Restoring Your Post-pregnancy Body, Naturally Using Women's Traditional Wisdom*. Kuala Lumpur, Malaysia: Percetakan Lenang Istimewa Sdn Bhd, 2012. Print.

Oakes, Ysha. "Ayurvedic Postpartum Care." *Ayurvedic Postpartum Care | Sacred Window School*. Sacred Window School: Ysha Oakes, n.d. Web. 05 Feb. 2016. <http://www.sacredwindow.com/>.

Romm, Aviva Jill. *Natural Health after Birth: The Complete Guide to Postpartum Wellness*. Rochester, VT: Healing Arts, 2002. Print.

# CHAPTER 6
## Building Your Postpartum Care Team

Gaskin, Ina May. "Ina May Gaskin." *Ina May Gaskin*. Inamay.com, 19 Sept. 2011. Web. 06 July 2016. <http://inamay.com/laureate-2011-right-livelihood-award/>.

Pascali Bonaro, Debra. "About - Debra Pascali Bonaro." *Debra Pascali Bonaro*. Debra Pascali Bonaro, n.d. Web. 30 Nov. 2016.

# Photo Credits

Cover Art: Tamara Adams, www.TamaraAdamsArt.com

Page 35, 52, 57, 59, 86: Jennifer Lind Schutsky, www.jenniferlindschutsky.com

Page 42, back cover bio image: Michelle Peterson

Page 47: © Milkos

Page 52: Sarah Carter

Page 53: Lorna Dufour

Page 72: © VadimGuzhva

Page 73: Danielle Haines, www.DanielleHaines.com

Page 80: © Olaf Speier | Dreamstime.com

Page 81, 102, 107: Shell Luttrell, www.MidwivesRising.com
www.ShellLuttrell.com

Page 83: © dglimages

Page 85, 86, 115: La Pachanga Photography, www.lapachangaphoto.com

Page 88: © JenkoAtaman

Page 89: © Ondras | Dreamstime.com

Page 92, 111: © Monkey Business

Page 99: Joy Winkleman, www.thegoodmedicineshop.com

Page 106: © contrastwerkstatt

93640909R00086

Made in the USA
San Bernardino, CA
09 November 2018